Living Normally with Dementia

One Care Home's Story
and How to Make It Yours

May Bjerre Eiby

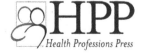

HPP
Health Professions Press

Baltimore • London • Sydney

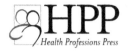

Health Professions Press, Inc.
Post Office Box 10624
Baltimore, Maryland 21285-0624

www.healthpropress.com

This is a translation from Danish to English of *Omsorgsmanifestet—Hvordan vi skaber verdens bedste plejehjem,* by May Bjerre Eiby in collaboration with Dorthe Boss Kyhn. Translation prepared by Solvej Scharling Todd.

Interior and Cover designs by Mindy Dunn
Typeset by Absolute Service, Inc., Towson, MD
Manufactured in the United States of America by Books International, Dulles, VA

The information provided in this book is in no way meant to substitute for the advice or opinion of a medical, legal, or other professional expert. Readers should consult a medical professional if they are interested in more information on dementia. This book is sold without warranties of any kind, express or implied, and the publisher and authors disclaim any liability, loss, or damage caused by the contents of this book.

Permission to print the photographs on the following pages is gratefully acknowledged: Cover photo and pages xxiv, xxvi, 1, 84, 110, 187, 198, and 199 (Liz Margerum); Frontispiece, pages 66, 165, and 221 (Per Fredrik Skiöld). We also thank the residents or their families for permission to include photos and stories of some of the residents of Dagmarsminde in this book. In most instances, names and identifying details have been changed to protect confidentiality. Real names and identifying details are used with permission.

Library of Congress Cataloging-in-Publication Data
Names: Eiby, May Bjerre, author.
Title: Living normally with dementia : one care home's story and how to
    make it yours / by May Bjerre Eiby
Other titles: Omsorgsmanifestet. English
Description: Baltimore : Health Professions Press, [2023]
    | Originally published in Danish as Omsorgsmanifestet: hvordan vi skaber
    verdens bedste plejehjem.
Identifiers: LCCN 2022037334 | ISBN 9781938870996 (paperback)
Subjects: LCSH: Dementia--Patients--Nursing home care. |
    Dementia--Patients--Nursing home care--Case studies. |
    Dementia--Patients--Long term care. | Medical personnel and patient.
Classification: LCC RC521 .E3313 2022 | DDC 616.8/310231--dc23/eng/20220831
LC record available at https://lccn.loc.gov/2022037334

British Library Cataloguing in Publication are available from the British Library.

Contents

———— ♦♦♦ ————

On the cover: Dagmarsminde resident Grete Lindberg, flight attendant, gym teacher, and mother of four, who always takes her tea with sugar and milk. (Photo: Liz Margerum)

About the Author

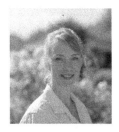

MAY BJERRE EIBY is a certified nurse with a master's degree in nursing from the University of Aarhus in Denmark. Most of her work has been with older adults in nursing homes and hospitals. In 2016, she established Dagmarsminde, a small nursing home north of Copenhagen for people with dementia. Her goal was to create a care home founded on more compassionate, person-centered practices than she had found in other care settings, especially for those with dementia. The approach to care at Dagmarsminde is built on a deep knowledge of each resident's needs and personalized care emphasizing comfort, individual attention, and active engagement of staff with both the residents and their relatives. In adopting this vision, the staff at Dagmarsminde have successfully eliminated the use of anti-psychotic medicines and sedatives and enabled their residents to live active, normal lives in the company of others.

Eiby has lectured around the world on the current state of dementia care and her distinctive approach to it. In 2021, in recognition of her efforts to challenge the status quo in elder care, she earned the prestigious Fonsmark Prize, awarded to a Danish citizen who helps raise public awareness. In addition, Dagmarsminde is the subject of the 2021 documentary directed by Louise Detlefsen, *It Is Not Over Yet.*

Foreword

———— •◆• ————

It has been more than a quarter century since the late Professor Tom Kitwood published his seminal work, *Dementia Reconsidered: The Person Comes First* (1997), in which he laid the groundwork for a more humane, holistic, and relational approach to care and support. In the years since, Kitwood's ideas have been widely adopted and evolved by academicians, and his concept of "person-centered care" has been touted by researchers and practitioners alike (a Google search of the term yields more than 300 million results).

Sadly, this vision is far from reality for most people living with the diagnosis in residential care homes around the world. In addition, the traditional pathology-centered biomedical view of dementia has informed practices that erode the well-being of people who live in the community as well as in congregate care settings.

The escalating number of people who are projected to develop dementia over the next few decades is often labeled a "tsunami"—an offensive term used to frame our evolving demographics as a tragedy in the making. But a far greater tragedy is that so many people will one day be relegated to lives devoid of meaning, comfort, and affirmation simply because there is no place for these in our dominant system of care.

Fortunately, out of the countless stories of lives lost to institutionalization, isolation, sedation, and restraint emerge people who have turned their personal tragedies into a passion to change the trajectory of what a life with dementia might become. May Bjerre Eiby is one of these people, and in Dagmarsminde she has created perhaps the most startling and life-affirming home for people living with dementia that I have ever seen. It is not a village, a fabricated environment, or a place rife with gadgets and artificial engagement platforms. It is simply a home that is guided by the notion that people with a diagnosis of dementia should be enabled to continue to live authentic, valued, and purposeful lives—a notion that is infused through every aspect of life in Dagmarsminde.

In this book, May bridges the frustrating gulf that often exists between philosophy and practice, sharing the nuts and bolts of daily life at Dagmarsminde. In doing so, she draws on several core concepts that are essential to transforming our approach to care and support for people living with a diagnosis of dementia.

First, there is a *deep commitment to normality* that reveals itself right up front in the table of contents. The chapters are built around various aspects of life and overall well-being rather than clinical categories, routines, symptoms, or care scenarios. A central tenet is learning each person's unique rhythms and letting these guide the manner in which the day unfolds instead of squeezing people who live with changing cognition into previously established and rigid routines.

But normality goes well beyond a daily schedule at Dagmarsminde. The ways in which people's adjustments to their environment, expressions, reactions, and emotions are looked upon as normal and legitimate human responses rather than "challenging behaviors" sets the stage for an entirely different set of assumptions, expectations, approaches, and ultimately, results. Normality informs all aspects of life in the home—in how residents are first welcomed, how they are encouraged to engage with the natural world, how traditional therapies are replaced by organic physical activities, and so much more. On the very first day the staff welcomes the new resident with mindful care.

Second, the commitment to normality for those who reside at Dagmarsminde means *acknowledging the person's view*

of the world and framing care approaches around it. This practice shows a deep respect for each person's right to see the
world through his or her own lens, validates these individual
perspectives, and offers support built around each person's
unique worldview, values, and preferences. For example, in
Chapter 3, May relates the story of a woman who was found
rummaging through her clothes and unable to get herself
washed and dressed. It is a perfect illustration of a mindset
that says, "You are okay, what you have done is not a problem,
and my task is to help you get 'unstuck' in ways that do not
demean you or threaten your self-esteem."

Third, like many transformative long-term care movements, Dagmarsminde places a primacy on *deep, continuous,
knowing relationships.* As such, this book sounds the call to
move away from generic protocols and interventions to deep
connection, empathy, and even clinical judgment that is guided by the instincts arising from this deep knowing. Relationships supersede generic "rules."

Flowing forth from these deep relationships are multiple
examples of how to view and engage in the important *minutiae
of everyday life.* This is not simply a book describing special
celebrations or "bucket list" initiatives. Rather, it highlights
the important knowledge that meaningful life grows most successfully when the myriad small moments of each day are infused with that same degree of meaning.

Another outgrowth of this care philosophy is the recognition that *an overabundance of fear can inform very dangerous
decisions* about design, technology, safety, and activity. Fear
can also lead to potentially harmful interpersonal interactions,
both verbal and nonverbal. The proof of rejecting fear-based
approaches lies in the real-life results that were evident during my 2017 visit to Dagmarsminde and that are still manifest
today: people whose condition and functional levels have stabilized or improved since moving in; joyous and enthusiastic
engagement, from dancing to a Tom Jones recording to singing hymns at a religious service; support without the use of

psychotropic medications; and, when people eventually enter their final days, engagement of the entire community in easing and celebrating their passing.

Lastly, this book shows the *power of creating true community* within the home, sharing empathy and coming together to help each other rather than reinforcing differences. The result of all of these mind shifts is the creation of a home that not only provides exceptional care, but also restores the sacredness of the work performed and the lives lived.

Even if you don't plan to build a home like Dagmarsminde, this book is an essential guide for seeing, caring for, and supporting people living with dementia; indeed, it is a guide for supporting people in any living environment—regardless of abilities—and celebrating our shared humanity.

G. Allen Power, M.D.
Rochester, New York, USA
September 18, 2022

Dr. Power is the author of *Dementia Beyond Drugs: Changing the Culture of Care* (© 2016; 2010) and *Dementia Beyond Disease: Enhancing Well-Being* (© 2017; 2014), published by Health Professions Press.

Preface

———◦◆◦———

WAITING IN THE HALL are a couple hundred leaders, investors, and directors from the Australian care home sector. They are attentively listening to the enthusiastic host introducing the audience to the next speaker at the conference. I smile nervously and try to look calm, while the host talks about the "Nordic nurse," who founded her own little nursing home, Dagmarsminde, in Denmark.

In a few minutes I'm going to speak in front of the crowd, and I suddenly wish I'd written something down, because I can't remember a word of it. My heart is hammering and I'm nauseous after the 10,000-mile trip, which included stops in Bergen and Tokyo to visit nursing homes and tell them about the type of care we offer at my nursing home for people with dementia.

I'm going to tell them about back then, back when we opened the doors and the first residents moved in and immediately showed signs of improvement. About the ones who lacked all motivation, but who stopped taking their medication, opened up to us, and regained some of their lost abilities, exclusively through the use of *care* as a treatment form. About distraught relatives who were reunited with their family member. About the media that reported our results of replacing medicine with human closeness. About the waiting list for Dagmarsminde, which within a few months became the longest in the country. About the residents we sat with as they exhaled their last breath. About the resistance from those in the public nursing home sector who claimed our methods were dangerous. About the hundreds of thousands on social media who saw our hand-held videos and pictures showing the transformation of our residents.

Jytte, who went from a wheelchair to walking up stairs. Henning, who suddenly communicated in whole sentences when we went jogging together. Kirsten, who participated in household activities, when 2 years before at another nursing home she had rarely left her room. About the many who shared their experiences of the awful conditions at care homes across the country and made us realize we hadn't just created a little nursing home; we'd created a counterculture. About the joy of touching trees and smelling the herbs in the garden. About preventing urinary tract infections and avoiding expensive hospitalizations. About serving restaurant food, and pampering on a daily basis, enabling a vulnerable elderly person to regain hope and self-esteem.

This is what I want to talk about, except I'm at a loss for words. How do you say "circadian rhythm" in English? "Care treatment"? My mind has gone blank, and it's too late to escape. I make my way through the hall and up to the podium. It's make or break.

When I founded Dagmarsminde in 2016, I wanted to create a place where people with severe dementia could receive high-quality personal care, the kind my family missed out on when my father developed dementia and wasted away in a corner of the county nursing home, before dying in 2013 due to an indifferent staff.

I was motivated to do better. I believed we had to fundamentally change the system, and so I decided to create my own nursing home. I'd been preparing for years, unknowingly at first. I earned a master's degree in nursing and, equipped with all sorts of theoretical ideas, naively believed I could make a difference within the public nursing sector. But then I ran into a wall of bureaucracy and stiff complacency from the bottom all the way up.

A little older, a little wiser, I turned my back on the public sector and focused on the writings of a Norwegian philosopher and professor of nursing science, Kari Martinsen, on nursing and caring for the vulnerable in our society. The Danish philosopher Knud Ejler Løgstrup's involuted book, *The Ethical Demand (Den Etiske Fordring)*, also helped me establish a view of human nature, where dependence is presented as fundamental and beneficial to care work. Today, this is one of the driving forces of the resident–staff relationship at Dagmarsminde.

As I write this, there are currently 12 residents at Dagmarsminde with severe dementia. They are my inspiration—it is their home. They are the vulnerable ones, who don't fit in anywhere else. They offer my fellow staff and me an abundance of knowledge on a daily basis. Although a lot of healthcare politicians like to use Dagmarsminde as a kind of showcase when trying to prove their dedication to the elderly population, we aren't actually used to receiving a lot of support from the Danish care sector—then again, we're not always so positive about the conditions at public nursing homes, either.

Outside of Denmark, the reception has not been quite as tentative. We have been met with enthusiasm from the start. Ever since I opened Dagmarsminde, I have been invited to give talks in more countries than I could have ever imagined; also, of course, for lots of inspiring audiences in Denmark, as well.

So here I am in Australia. At the podium at a conference in Sydney, where I have completely forgotten the nursing terminology in English, and the audience is following my every move in anticipation. I take a deep breath and remember my mother, who always had a way of breaking the ice with her sense of humor. "I'm very thankful to be here today. Some of you who visited my little nursing home in Denmark know my English isn't very good. So, if you'll bear with me, I'll take it in Danish from here." The audience bursts into laughter. We're on the same page now, luckily. My pulse returns to normal. The English words that had momentarily escaped me have returned.

People with all types of dementia struggle on a daily basis to conceal their lost abilities from the "normal" outside world, and they do exactly the same thing as I did at the podium. They compensate by diverting their surroundings from their diminishing capacities and their incomprehension by blurting out something funny, redirecting the conversation, or nodding to the person across from them, while in reality their words are lost in a mumbling fog.

As the illness advances, it becomes increasingly difficult to maintain the illusion of fitting into the regular social circles of family, work, or friends. The contexts that constitute one's life are gradually limited, a situation that would be grievous for anyone, because no one likes losing their sense of worth or can stand feeling lost every second of every day. The moment arrives when the illusion bursts, and there is no more denying that the person with dementia cannot take care of themselves anymore. So, he or she is brought to a nursing home, which for many is the beginning of a sad downward spiral, and for reasons that I will explain in later chapters becomes a kind of waiting room for death.

It's time for a radical change—both in Denmark and other countries—because the care sector is stuck, and has been for decades. In Denmark, it is vulnerable elders who are paying the price for the resigned panic running through the whole disenchanted health sector, with its focus on salaries, medicating, help aids, time off, and constant complaining about the care one is employed to do. In the U.S. and other countries, these elders suffer due to societal constraints resulting in overworked, low-paid care partners; one-size-fits-all care standards; and ageism.

There Is an Alternative

I cannot count the number of times I've heard it's impossible to create a fantastic care home—that there isn't enough money, there aren't enough caring souls, the work is too strenuous, the elderly are too sick, the pay is too low, the set-up is all wrong, there's not enough light, there's not enough room, and that the world's best nursing home is only for the wealthy.

I have only one thing to say: It's a grand misconception. It's an argument borne out of a world gone astray. One where we've forgotten our innate obligation to look out for one another. Where we've forgotten the most important cornerstone of our culture, of our families: the elderly. We've forgotten how to navigate in this world without rigidly relying on models, recommendations, manuals, data, and what others are doing. Our intuition has been eradicated by a desperate search for something that gives us a clear result, a clear answer or an outcome, without us having to discern, decide, or engage.

We no longer believe in our own abilities. There is no point in a world where things are only taken seriously if they have been proved and tested. Working in this kind of environment eliminates any motivation to change things, or to believe we can create a fantastic nursing home. But we can.

Living Normally with Dementia is my best bid for what a care home can be if we want to be proud of our care sector. We can create the world's best nursing homes, whether they are paid for by the residents or the state. Most of the residents at Dagmarsminde live on a standard pension, and our care home receives the same financial support from the state as any other nursing home within the Danish welfare state.

Dagmarsminde is not the world's best nursing home yet, but we're working on it. I hope our experiences will motivate you to think and act differently in your daily interactions with elders affected by dementia. Together we can create the world's best elder care if we want to.

As you read on, you will be introduced to a way of thinking about care and nursing that may inspire you to create a more normal and meaningful life for the residents at your care home. My readings of K. E. Løgstrup and Kari Martinsen, along with texts on traditional nursing rooted in Christian values, have shaped my approach. I want to prove that nursing theory and philosophy can be put into practice. That is the extent to which this book is academic. I make a point of liberating myself from the confines of science, research objectivity, and so on. Citing sources is not part of my daily work. I'm grateful to the people who have inspired me, but readers will notice that I don't cite them here. The sources and their followers will recognize when I've incorporated their words into my work. I've already mentioned the most significant ones. Everything I've written here is an amalgam of my readings and my hands-on experience.

I describe the work I do and my ideas on care and nursing. It is entirely based on my experiences from Dagmarsminde, where my staff and I care for the most vulnerable elderly population, namely those with dementia. This book is intended for anyone close to a person with dementia, whether you are a professional or a relative. It is an example of how to run a nursing home for dementia, but it is applicable to all types of care homes.

Organization of This Book

The book follows daily life at our nursing home, from a resident's first day to his or her very last breath. I have divided the book into three phases: Part I, The Rehabilitating and Stabilizing Phase; Part II, The Weakening Phase; and Part III, The Final Phase. Along the way, I have included specific stories of life at Dagmarsminde, as well as some accounts from relatives.

I examine a number of key turning points and everyday acts of care in our work with the residents, showing how we use care as a form of treatment on a daily basis. It is important to break free from the way most care homes are run today, which I describe in the sections titled "The Norm." It is no secret that I hear a lot of excuses for why we cannot improve things. I counter these in the sections titled "Objection."

I have written this book both to encourage and to challenge you to reform your nursing home. Whether that means planting more trees in the garden or listening to and learning from the way a resident breathes or creating a relaxing shared space with natural light, I look forward to hearing about it.

Acknowledgments

I extend my gratitude and appreciation to the many people who contributed in their own ways to the creation of this book:

- To the residents who currently reside and have resided at Dagmarsminde and their families

- To my staff, who work hard for the residents everyday—day, evening, and night

- To my eternally loyal sparring partner and fellow traveler, Dorte

- To all the relatives and the health professionals I have met along the way

- To Kari Martinsen, for her words and her strike of lightning, for understanding our approach, and for giving the field of nursing greater purpose and meaning

- To Carl Austin Hyatt, for sparring and inspiration on the chapters regarding nature and energies

- To my beloved, Carl Jonas, for reading and feedback on my texts and for your trust and faith in my vision

- To my family, my four children, and their father

Introduction to Dagmarsminde

A Care Oasis

———— •◆• ————

DAGMARSMINDE IS A SMALL NURSING HOME with 12 residents, all of whom have severe dementia. New residents usually come to us from other nursing homes—places unable to meet their needs. Others have moved directly from their own homes.

The condition of our newly arrived residents is no different from those moving in at other nursing homes. Some are in a weakened physical state upon arrival, their mobility having been limited by the use of a wheelchair or lift, while others can still move around freely. Being more mobile, however, does not necessarily mean being less cognitively challenged than those in a wheelchair. And while each faces challenges of his or her own, they all require care around the clock. They cannot make it on their own.

Therapeutic care at Dagmarsminde consists of three main components: care, aesthetics, and tapering residents off all forms of medication. This means the staff do not administer any calming or antipsychotic drugs. On the contrary, in collaboration with the home's general practitioner, they gradually reduce the resident's long list of daily medications. Once the medicine no longer masks the resident's actual symptom picture, with its side effects and adverse ramifications, new possibilities open for the staff to engage and reach the resident. The care treat-

Dagmarsminde: Inside and Out

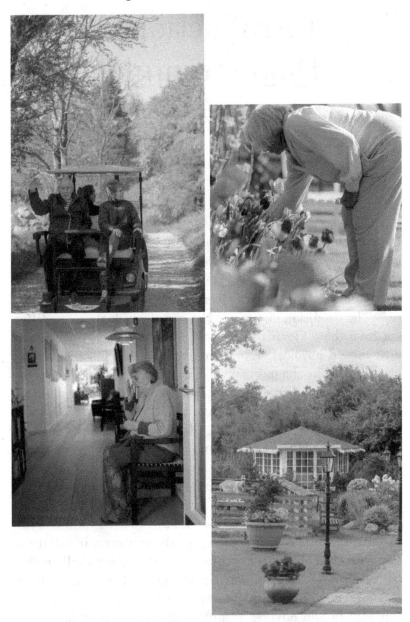

ment is based on establishing trust, acknowledgment, touch, and encouraging physical activity and mental stimuli. Most of this work occurs within the home's shared spaces and with the fellowship of our community. The residents are together from morning until evening, constantly supported by a schedule and stable routine that is mindful of their needs and repeats every day. The environment surrounding the residents and the staff is carefully orchestrated to ensure a calm and peaceful atmosphere. It feels and looks like a real home, without a hint of a workplace.

The number of employees on site is 2.5 at all times: two in the evening and two at night. Occasionally a third staff member comes in as needed, but only for a portion of the day. Each day shift includes one trained nurse and sometimes one during the night shifts too. Additionally, there is always a nurse on call, whom the staff can contact for advice, and who can be there within the hour. The employees who are not nurses include health assistants and carers, both trained and untrained, as well as health professionals who have switched from a different area within healthcare. We do not require fixed sets of skills for these employees. Our focus is on their human skills coupled with a demonstrated competence in relating to our residents and staff. Training employees in our methods and values is an ongoing and constant process.

A detailed layout of our grounds appears on page xxvii, after this Introduction. Dagmarsminde has three large connected shared spaces: a communal dining area, an openplan kitchen, and an adjacent rest area. There are also 10 resident rooms, each with its own ergonomic bath and toilet. Two of these rooms are used by couples. Five of the rooms have direct access to the terrace and garden. Dagmarsminde also has a small spa area with a warm-water therapy pool and a cozy reading room. The garden around the house is enclosed by a fence, allowing the residents to walk around on their own without the risk of wandering off. It is filled with flowers and herbs, tiny pathways, and calming spaces to sit and relax. Our garden is used year round.

Not far from Dagmarsminde is a forest where the staff often take walks with the residents. We have two golf carts that the staff sometimes use to take residents on a scenic drive through the trees. Creating a connection to the natural world around us is at the core of our work.

I describe Dagmarsminde as a "care oasis" because the care home is the kind of place the residents needed throughout all those years when their disease developed and they were weighed down by obstacles such as overmedication, being stigmatized by society, and struggling with language and feelings of emptiness and failure. When they move to Dagmarsminde, it should feel like an oasis, a place delivering them from their arduous journey. They are met by warmth, professionalism, and an appreciation of who they are. From there on, they slowly and calmly regain their integrity as the daily framework of the final stage of their lives is shaped by a normalizing and supportive environment.

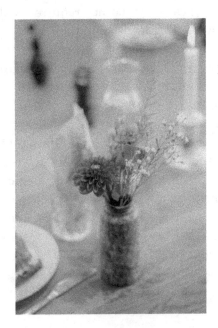

Dagmarsminde Buildings and Grounds

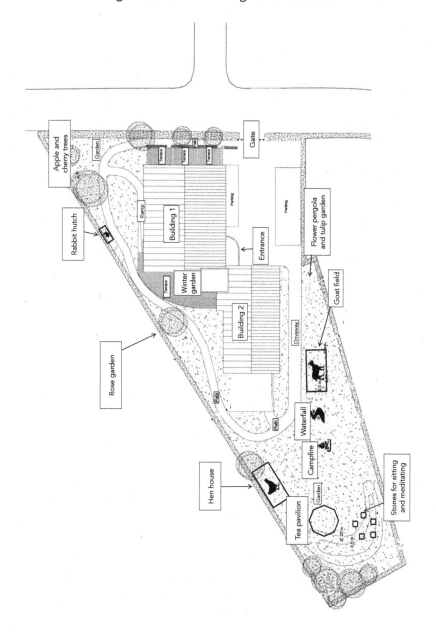

PART ONE

The Rehabilitating and Stabilizing Phase

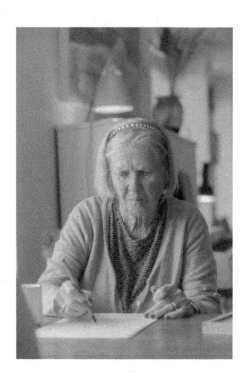

1

The Move

Crossing the Threshold to a New Life

A NURSING HOME SHOULD PROVIDE proper care for a person, but it can also be a place that opens up new possibilities. What if moving to a nursing could become a kind of adventure for people? Our goal at Dagmarsminde is to make moving to a nursing home a normal, even nice, experience for new residents.

Entering a New Life

The new resident is still the teacher, man, woman, parent, and grandparent he or she always was; the person's identity does not disappear upon moving to a nursing home. The transition to the nursing home must be accomplished with the utmost care and respect for the person moving in and for who they are. A good mantra for anyone working in the care sector is this: Let new residents sense they are welcome from the moment they arrive, even if they are old and affected by dementia.

We try very hard to put ourselves in the residents' shoes. New residents are on the threshold of the final phase of life. They cannot take care of themselves at home anymore, or they have just left a different nursing home because they did not receive the care they needed there.

Let new residents sense they are welcome from the moment they arrive, even if they are old and affected by dementia.

In preparing for the new resident, staff members make time to talk with the person's loved ones. We try to find out who the person is, and what is important to him or her. We want to know about our new resident's work life, interests and hobbies of the past and present, and any important life milestones. We also ask about the effect that dementia has had on the person and how he or she is doing at this time.

Before the resident's arrival, we place a welcome basket on the windowsill with flowers, chocolate, some snacks, a bottle of non-alcoholic wine or lemonade, and a little card with a personal note. We write that we are looking forward to getting to know them and having them be a part of our lives. We have pre-stocked the bathroom with lotion, shampoo, fingernail clippers, toothpaste, and a toothbrush. Even if they bring their own toiletries, we are signaling to both the new resident and the family that we have everything covered. There is no need for anyone to run around at the last minute buying forgotten everyday supplies.

Most relatives are worried about the move. They assume it is better to slowly phase in their loved one by having the person visit the place a couple of times in advance. They also think they have to move all the furniture and prepare the room beforehand. However, at Dagmarsminde, we do everything on the same day. We have tried different models and time frames, but this way actually seems the least disruptive, even when boxes, nervous relatives, and an often confused new resident all arrive at the same time.

This approach works because we make sure it is well coordinated; each staff member has a specific role or set of responsibilities during the move, and takes care to adhere to them throughout the day. One staff member welcomes and stays with the resident while the move is in progress. Another presents the room and helps carry and arrange things if needed, staying nearby and talking to the relatives, who are often so distraught by the situation that they do not always hear what we say. Our primary concern is that they feel that everything is in order and that we are honored to receive their loved one.

It is important to understand that a new resident's life has already been dramatically affected by dementia and he or she has usually suffered considerable hardship. The person has likely lost many basic abilities. Some need a wheelchair to move around, and others have lost the ability to speak. As a result of medications they have been given, they may have mentally shut down or be disoriented and anxious. A new resident may be on high alert and stressed—another reason to ensure the move is as seamless as possible. The shift from one world to another can feel very intense for a new resident.

While all the furniture gets carried in, the new resident is introduced to our shared living room. At first we do not invite the person to sit among the others; instead, the staff member guides him or her to a cozy space in the room for a quiet chat. We do not want to overload the resident with information. In these chats we will usually just talk about the weather and other trivial subjects. We give the person time to size us up and take in his or her surroundings. Throughout this time, the staff member maintains eye contact and remembers to smile. We might also invite the new resident to take a little walk in the garden; a little fresh air usually works wonders.

New residents generally have no interest in moving to a nursing home. This is one of the reasons we do not refer to it as a permanent move, and if they ask what they are doing here, we say they are here for a while to recuperate, exercise, get their bearings, or have a nice time with some fun people. We try to align with that person's self-perception and what he or she feels a need for here and now. Putting things this way often reassures the resident. If it does not work, we have to distract the person as well as we can with short walks, keeping up a lively conversation and avoiding anxiety-provoking empty silences.

We allow for all types of reactions from the residents. During these first hours, it is important to help minimize the stress level of the person to avoid having the transition become a traumatic experience for either the resident or members of the family. If the person tires of all our questions and walks, we suggest a little rest. By that time the bed and room are usually ready. Once the person sees his or her room filled with familiar things and senses the presence of family, the situation usually improves.

After the Loved Ones Leave

When the relatives leave, sometimes the residents do not understand the situation they are in. They may become sad and try to find the front door. "What is this place. . .?" The feeling of emptiness and fear is only natural. At this point new residents might start pacing back and forth. For some, the reaction is more pronounced than for others, but it is all perfectly normal. We give them some space, keep an eye on them, and then see what happens as—slowly but surely—the resident becomes a part of our community.

Later in the afternoon of the very first day, we introduce the resident and talk about his or her interests with the others at a little celebration with coffee and cake. The residents are always welcoming toward the new person, and after only a few days we usually start to see a transformation.

Even in the most complicated cases, being acknowledged by the entire household has a positive effect on the residents. They sense this is a place where there is always someone ready to help and happy to listen to their frustrations, and who does not react if they make a mistake.

Gradually, the resident relaxes. The staff are attentive, listening, and caring. Within the first few days, they pick up on the resident's patterns, interests, and ways of communicating; they chart his or her daily rhythms; and they are even able to ascertain a suitable amount of activity and rest for the person. With all of this careful attention, along with good food, adequate liquid, touch, and physical activity, the person's expression softens. After a few weeks, the new resident feels more at ease because their needs are met and because they sense they have come to a place where they can be themselves. The person is not just a resident at a nursing home but is someone who is living a long life.

Communicating with the New Resident

Many new residents can be frustrated and want to talk about the move or something else in their life that feels difficult. The staff need to listen and identify with these frustrations. In the beginning, our approach could be described as "motherly," or as a compassionate authority. For example, if a resident is having trouble understanding why he or she has been moved to a home, a care partner might say, "Well, you're here now, and I understand you think that's strange. But while you're here, we're going to do our best to make you happy. I'm always here to talk with you if you're having a hard time."

Residents almost never ask about the actual time frame of their stay; perhaps it is simply too abstract. We utilize this inability to grasp abstract concepts when things get too difficult for them. We are obviously not being completely truthful with them, but there is nothing wrong with telling them they are going to be here for a while. Of course, we are always mindful about lying because it can lead to distrust. Establishing trust between staff and resident is paramount.

What often bothers the residents most when they first move in is an all-consuming suspicion of almost everyone around. This often happens when residents come from other nursing homes where they have experienced neglect. In these cases, it can take several months for a resident to trust us. Once we get that far, we slowly work on getting the resident to open up to us—it takes time to get acquainted. For some, we can talk about their move from day one, but very few ever truly grasp that the nursing home is now their permanent home. It is not unusual for some residents to never fully comprehend it, and for years to refer to their stay as a little time away for some rest and relaxation. In any case, once they feel comfortable, they do not want to leave.

A couple of days after they arrive, most new residents start showing signs of improvement. The change for the better is significant for both the person with dementia and the relatives, who may see for example that their loved one actually *can* feed him- or herself and is eating with others without needing help. Or a new resident might suddenly try to formulate a whole sentence because he or she senses we are willing to wait for the words to come. We respond not only by talking, but with our eyes and with touch if the person cannot find the words to finish a sentence. Every positive experience, even the tiniest improvement, helps whet the appetite for both the resident and the staff member. The person's improved self-esteem has a domino effect. They feel that everything is going to be fine, so change is on the way.

Understanding Dementia

Dementia is the only terminal condition in which the person with the disease believes he or she is getting better. It can seem like a catastrophe for those who do not have it more than for the person who has been diagnosed. This is not to say that a person with dementia is not facing some tough personal challenges on a daily basis. People with dementia are obviously distressed when they cannot communicate or take care of themselves. Yet despite this distress, the person often perceives him- or herself as less and less "afflicted" as time passes. For us at Dagmarsminde, it is a source of inspiration.

Working with the Resident's Perception

We closely follow the residents and their individual experience of the dementia, so we can better identify with their situation and try to meet their needs. Of course, sometimes that means having to take corrective actions to prevent accidents. But we do not have to correct every mistake or misunderstanding. Sometimes we have to let the residents do things that seem strange to the rest of us—for instance, putting their teacup down under a plant in our garden. But who is to say they are not onto something? They have momentarily stepped into another reality, and it is our job to step back.

At other times, we might need to steer the resident toward a more realistic perception, but we have to do this subtly so he or she does not notice that we have we have negated the person's previous perception. For example, a resident may be afraid of taking a bath. From the resident's perspective, it might feel like an invasion of his or her privacy, and be intimidating, when a staff member suddenly asks the person to take off their clothes or just starts undressing the resident. This can be difficult even if the staff member has explained the process and is careful. Before and during the bath, we can divert the person's anxiety by first letting the warm water run down his or her back for a little time while we describe how nice it must be to feel the warm water on one's back, and that it is a nice day and we are going to take a walk in the sunshine together.

Life at Our Home

One of our residents likes to collect other residents' clothes in the laundry room where they're drying on hangers. She believes she has been shopping and proudly shows us her new shirts when she comes into the living room. Then, sometimes suddenly, the activity gets out of hand. She gets confused and stressed about all her "purchases." We try to keep her focused on the clothes she's already "bought." We ask her to hang them up in her closet (where we will retrieve them when she isn't looking), and then we lock the laundry room while she does that. It is an invisible rectification of her reality. The day is often a balancing act between recognizing the resident's reality and acknowledging it, followed by our invisible correction.

Our approach is all about respecting the resident's perception of normality, especially if it means preserving the optimism that exists in not knowing one has a brain disease. We try, so to speak, to understand the illness from *the resident's* understanding of having dementia or not—whether the person sees his or her behavior as normal or not. The resident's perception is the gauge for what is "normal." Some experts may claim that this is a risky way of dealing with a condition such as dementia, because the healthy person "knows best." We are trying to turn this way of thinking around. Working with people who have dementia is mainly about the healthy person's openness toward the behavior and experience of the person

Life at Our Home

One of our residents sometimes feels the need to put things inside his shirt. There is no limit to the number of things he can carry—a crime novel, three washcloths, all the remote controls from our shared living room, my iPhone, and my colleague's glasses. One day, I watched him pass through our kitchen, where I had left out a juice box on the counter. He quickly picked it up and put in his pocket. As we got to know him better, we realized this behavior was a sign of inner turmoil. Now we help him by not letting him get to the point where he needs to collect things. Once we curbed this behavior by anticipating his restlessness and stimulating him with, among other things, long walks, conversations about his family pictures, and coordination exercises, he became a whole other person. His sentence construction improved and he opened up to other residents more—in his own way.

We also have him help clean up the kitchen, entirely at his leisure. In fact, he has concluded that *we* are the ones staying at *his* house. This conclusion is a sign of stabilizing perception—the resident has made sense, in his own way, of the situation—a code we cracked because we viewed the restless collecting behavior as more than just a symptom of the disease. It was merely a creative and unique way of telling us he needed help and more stimulation.

with dementia. This approach also involves openness toward what is acceptable and can be classified as normal, and shows how people with dementia can harmoniously coexist with those who do not have dementia.

We try to create a fun, inspiring, and creative community with the residents. In fact, they are an uplifting bunch! Once in a while, there are challenges, as when a person yells, strikes out, or is restless, but for the most part it is a positive environment because people with dementia live in the present. They feel healthy and not as old as their age would indicate. They can benefit from that. Imagine having the firm belief that you were never old or sick!

I am often amazed by the creativity of my residents, both in their sudden impulses and in their ways of communicating. They make connections most of us would never imagine, and they experience the world in a way that inspires those of us who witness it.

Understanding Patterns of Behavior

People with dementia can feel themselves losing control more often than healthy people would. Many of their actions are a sign of their wanting to manage this loss, and each person's pattern or system of actions and expressions is unique. They may repeat sentences or actions or use specific terms or patterns to help them exist or cooperate with others. Some of these patterns may be more inappropriate than others; if there are many such patterns, it can be a sign of a hidden frustration we will need to address and mitigate.

We try to replace inappropriate patterns, such as moving furniture around, wearing several shirts, and so on, with more useful ones, such as adding certain activities within the set daily program, which I will elaborate upon later. Basically, working with a person with dementia means helping the person lessen the experience of having lost control. As the person without dementia, the care partner must be conscious of his or her own tolerance of the person's expressions.

Do you understand how residents perceive their condition, for example that they are not sick but are healthy and younger than their age? This is the usual self-perception of people with severe dementia. We can accomplish a lot by simply acknowledging their experience of the disease. This includes stepping back from the diagnosis and not using it as the basis for their treatment.

Focusing on the dementia diagnosis limits our understanding of the person sitting across from us. Regardless of the amount of information we read about the brain's systems and patterns, it does not compare to what we can perceive with a few seconds of eye contact. We never openly refer to a diagnosis at Dagmarsminde. This enables us to connect on a more human level—yet another reason the residents do not feel objectified, excluded, or unwanted.

We know the residents have dementia and that is enough. From the moment they pass through our doors, our focus is on being there for these people who need us. As you read this book, I invite you to put aside everything you know about the brain's functions or the pathology of certain types of dementia, because from here on, it is not needed.

The Norm: Welcome to the Care Home?

As noted at the beginning of this chapter, the arrival day is utterly crucial because it signifies the start of a new phase in life. A passive welcome matches the underlying reality of a dysfunctional environment. When management does not prioritize an arrival, it is a clear sign that they do not care who the new resident is. To them, the person has become an anonymous nursing home resident—no longer a homemaker, engineer, or piano teacher.

It is almost the rule rather than the exception that moving to a nursing home feels like a move into a scary unknown. The resident and the relative are left in the dark and feel neither comfortable nor welcome within the new setting. What they often feel instead is disregard.

A Relative's Experience

Here is an account from a resident's daughter:

When the move-in day arrived, we drove my mother to the nursing home. She was so happy, and she was really looking forward to it. At least that's what she said. I've often wondered if she thought she was moving back to her childhood home. My mother didn't know where she was, even after we arranged her new room with her furniture, pictures, and lamps.

We weren't allowed to bring her own bed. Instead she had a hospital bed with hospital sheets. We were told she had to use it. It never crossed my mind that my mother shouldn't have had a hospital bed. I just figured this was how it was when you moved to a nursing home.

It was a Sunday afternoon. A staff worker came into my mother's room with coffee and some cake. My mother sat in her armchair. She didn't say much, just sipped her coffee and ate her cake. We were alone. No one came in and gave us any information. After a while my mother got tired and slumped over in her chair.

I didn't know what to do. I went down to the staff in the shared living room and asked about the schedule. They told me I could leave and they would take it from there. I went back to my mother, who by this time, was fast asleep in her chair. As I drove home that day I had a bad feeling about it. I didn't know what the next days would bring, but I knew my mother would be upset when she woke up and discovered I was gone. I didn't sleep that night.

The next day I called the unit and asked how things were going. The staff worker sounded surprised. "Oh, everything's great," she said. When I went to see my mother later that afternoon, she was asleep in the reception hall, slumped face-down on the dining table.

There was no one around I could ask about my mother's first day. It took about half a year before the staff scheduled a meeting with me about my mother's move. I've never felt so alone. I felt like I'd let my mother down.

From Accomplished Engineer to Just Another Resident

Sven was a proud engineer who had spent his life building bridges—big, complicated steel constructions. Even though he had developed dementia and was moved to a nursing home, he still loved talking about his work. He was proud of the gigantic infrastructure projects he had been a part of. Unfortunately, the staff in his normal nursing home seemed uninterested in his past endeavors.

Sven's dementia obscured his memory like passing gray clouds. He was also hindered by poor hearing. He became increasingly isolated. In the end, he gave up. He could not handle being with the others in the living room. One day he fell and broke his hip, and for a couple of weeks he was in and out of the hospital. Ten days after he returned to the nursing home for the last time, he died.

Sven's story is only one of many in my inbox that illustrate the apparent indifference of many nursing home staff and what happens when people are left to oblivion and stripped of an identity. It is a symptom of a dysfunctional environment, apparent from day one, when a resident enters a nursing home and is not properly welcomed.

Consider the story of Karl, and see if any of it seems familiar. Karl lived in a nursing home for many years. Imagine him sitting in a corner of his room for hours on end, staring at the walker placed in front of him that has a basket full of napkins, an apple, and an incontinence pad. On the seat is a plastic sippy cup filled with a watery, lukewarm, red juice. Karl feels hot, as if he has a fever, but the staff tell him he is not sick. The metallic taste in his mouth keeps getting worse, and his ears are ringing. His skin feels prickly and itchy. His feet hurt, especially where his toenail is jammed in his shoe. He does not recognize the clothes he is wearing, and when he looks around the room he is not sure what he is doing there. Nearby is a bed with electrical cords and railings attached to it. Is this some sort of prison or psychiatric ward?

The days, weeks, and months pass without visitors. Karl has plenty of time to make himself comfortable, but all this time without activity is only making him more anxious. Is he who he thinks he is? His head is swimming with questions. What is the point anymore? He hates the people who come bursting into his room and shout at him. They sound weird and he never sees their eyes. They are not welcome anymore. Karl has bad breath. He only eats yogurt and drinks a couple glasses of the lukewarm juice, and he spits at the staff members when they come in with their loud voices and grim faces. He protests as much as he can. Mostly he stays in his bed. Strangely worn out and unhappy, he cries without tears. The last thing Karl hears at the end of his long life is someone saying: "Geeze, take a look. Could you bring a mop?"

Relief for the Relatives?

Many relatives fight a losing battle for their family member with dementia. For the relatives, the person who just moved into a nursing home is a father, a mother, a husband, or a wife with a life and with inherent value. It is painful to stand by and watch as a loved one loses his or her identity first to dementia and then to an institutionalized approach to care in a nursing home.

In order to change things, we have to start from the beginning, from day one, when a resident moves in. By this point the relatives are exhausted. They have usually been caring for their loved one at home and everything has been on their shoulders for years. Although they might have had home care help, the relatives have generally managed the daily routines. Or, the new resident might be coming from a nursing home where he or she experienced neglect—and where once again, the relatives have had to step in, advocate for the person, and, when that was not enough, arrange for their loved one to move to this new home.

Another reason the relatives are so exhausted is that their loved one is not the person they once knew, and the unfamiliar behavior can be unsettling to them. Relatives are often physically and mentally on the brink of collapse when their loved one finally arrives at a nursing home. They need to know the person they care about is comfortable within the new setting. They need peace and quiet to grieve, to reflect, to find new meaning. But their worry lingers. The relative keeps thinking about his or her loved one. *Is she lying on her side in her bed with her hand under her cheek, staring vacantly into the room? Is she alone at the dining table, chewing on a piece of bread? Is she thinking about the time I was a little girl playing on the beach in the summer? Or when she met my father? Is she sad he's not there with his arms around her? She doesn't know he's dead.* For family members who care for their loved ones, these concerns can be unbearable.

All of the existential questions and deliberations connected to this kind of crisis are too often pushed aside by the relatives' immediate concerns over whether their loved one will experience reproach, rough handling, the side effects of drugs, or simply indifference. Our current world of care work is often steered by "protocol" and charts, tracking the staff's tasks—or more specifically, keeping track of what the staff are doing. The entire care sector is dominated by this kind of mechanistic artifice, beginning with the resident's move into the home.

Objection:
"We'll have plenty of time to get acquainted."

When I have talked to staff from other nursing homes about their procedure for new arrivals, I seldom get the impression they have thought it over. The staff say they "welcome the resident," but when asked about the specific details or how they have decided what to do, the response is that it is different from one resident to the next.

Some things should not be left to chance or to how members of the team feel on a given day. The person's transition into the life of the nursing home should be thoroughly considered and carefully coordinated. Everything has to go smoothly. It is important to decide what the first impression should be for the resident and for his or her relatives. If our care home really means something to us, and we are proud of it, then we have to make the effort to present it as well as possible.

When I try to explain this to staff members from other nursing homes, some get irritated. Some will argue that the move-in does not influence the rest of a resident's stay. It is a separate process, and they get to know the resident later. But if the resident's first impression of the new home is one of either chaos or impersonal treatment, moving day will represent a new trauma for people who have already experienced a great deal of it.

Summary

It is an enormous upheaval for a vulnerable person to move into an unfamiliar place and begin having to engage with six or eight strangers every day. We should all do our utmost to welcome a new resident and to let the person know that we are looking forward to getting to know him or her.

Dementia remains a low-status condition. People with dementia do not fit the usual healthcare mold. It is not presently curable. We in the care sector can help to make things better—more person-centered and open to the person's reality and to helping him or her continue to thrive, even with dementia. We begin by welcoming them, whole-heartedly and with extreme care, to their new home.

———•◆•———

Questions for Reflection

1. Consider the practices of your organization with regard to the move-in of a new resident. What role do you play in the process? How long does it take?

2. What are some challenges and obstacles you and your colleagues face when introducing a new resident to your care home? Do you have ideas or suggestions for overcoming them?

3. How does the move-in process affect the resident's process of integrating into life at your home?

2

◦◆◦

Aesthetics

Balancing the Mind with Décor

PEOPLE WITH DEMENTIA MAY HAVE lost the ability to talk and their rational understanding of the world, but, in my experience, as their vulnerability increases, their sensitivity to external stimuli skyrockets, causing them to become unstable and more intense. When we stimulate the residents' senses in a good way, we lay the foundation for a balanced life of overall well-being. This is a large part of the work we do at Dagmarsminde.

The interior design of a nursing home should give the people using the space a feeling of belonging. This is especially important with regard to those with dementia who are moving to a new home. They are usually in a difficult phase of their illness and are less capable of managing assaults on their senses than others may be; they are dependent on others to create a comfortable space around them. The physical space can help the resident put the feeling of chaos, emptiness, and unfamiliarity behind them, allowing them to regain their sense of calm, stability, and connection. We can use the design to meet the resident's need to be led away from their suffering.

Surroundings and mood can function as a kind of communication between the resident and the people around them. It is increasingly clear to me that our residents are more open to our affection and care in spaces created with consideration for their sensing. We have designed the nursing home's spaces in a way that resonates with the residents' moods and helps them feel they belong here. We have to be "production designers" of the nursing home's spaces, setting the scene for well-being and relaxation, down to the smallest detail.

> *The interior design of a nursing home should give the people using the space a feeling of belonging.*

The Elements of Décor

It is helpful to consider all of the impressions we might experience within a single room: sounds, colors, temperature, and lighting; the scent we pick up on when we step in the door; the memory sparked by a piece of furniture from our childhood; the weight of a coffee cup in our hand; or fresh flowers. Sensory experiences let us know if a room is safe, whether we can relax or should be on the alert.

Working with Sound

The first element to consider when creating a more caring aesthetic at a nursing home is the acoustics. Although a room is quiet, it still has a sound, which either evokes discomfort or comfort, unease or calm, nervousness or certainty. This is caused by the room's reflection of sound waves.

We have all probably walked around a house without furniture, carpets, or household items to absorb the sound of our voice and our footsteps. Empty rooms without sound barriers have an eerie echo. We may have dined at a cafeteria without any sound insulation, where the noise got worse as those eating tried to make themselves heard. It is much nicer to enter a room that is cozy, warm, and atmospheric, such as an old library filled with books or a living room furnished with heavy carpets and soft furniture that absorb the sounds of talk and activity. We are not always conscious of it, but the sound quality of a room affects our well-being. That is why we try to stay aware of the acoustics throughout our nursing home. We have found people with dementia need sounds to be dampened.

Sound insulation can be expensive, but it is definitely something to consider if you are renovating. When sound is dampened, the air feels soft or "smooth." Noise is generally bothersome for most of us, but it can be literally uncomfortable for people with dementia, whose senses are already working at full capacity. Healthy people's senses are working too of course, but with dementia, one sense might be heightened while another is slightly muted. It can be very difficult to accommodate for the sudden overflow of input. The heart rate increases and the person can become anxious and stressed. Remember, people with dementia are already stressed when moving to a nursing home because life has become a constant challenge.

At Dagmarsminde, we have sound-insulated the floors, walls, and ceiling as in a recording studio. Sound does not carry between the rooms or floors. The sound-insulating material makes the air feel soft and calm. Almost everyone who visits says the same thing about stepping through our doors: "I let down my shoulders." This is the power of good acoustics.

Music has a huge effect on the mood in a room. It can function as a backdrop, which can magically absorb sudden metallic sounds like the clatter of cutlery or the "white noise" of a group of people talking over each other. We have high-quality loudspeakers placed in different locations, and we have compiled playlists to suit a wide variety of moods. In the morning, we often play quiet guitar or other instrumental music throughout the home. In our spa area, residents can enjoy the subtle chirping of birds, whale songs, and Zen tones. If a different mood is needed, we can choose from our list of piano sonatas, easy New Orleans jazz, or classics that were popular during our residents' earlier lives. The music has to match the atmosphere and the activity, and sometimes we have to try different styles to find the right one. We are constantly considering individual residents along with the group as a whole, checking to see if the atmosphere is as intimate as intended.

We never just leave the music blasting in the rooms because that would be unsettling for the residents. We turn up the volume if we are all going to dance, but at all other times we keep the music so low we can barely hear the words to a song. While the music is on, we have to stay alert and ready to adjust the sound level if a saxophone or a singer gets too lively or loud. A respectful handling of music can make a room come together, and we like our residents to pick up on that feeling of togetherness.

Life at Our Home

As noted, we often have music playing quietly in the background to create a comfortable atmosphere in the living room. But music can also serve a more specific function, such as helping us to transition between activities. The residents might have come back from the garden, and we want them to gather for our shared reading. Some of them will sit promptly down in the sofa, whereas others need a little help with their coats, going to the bathroom, and so on. The waiting time before the next activity tends to cause a bit of restlessness in the living room. Some residents may not really understand what they are waiting for—only that there is a shared event in the sofa area. It can easily take up to half an hour for everyone to find their places around the reader. In the meantime, if we play some familiar melodies and songs sung by the Danish National Girls' Choir and turn up the volume, it usually has a calming effect on the residents in the room. A few will sit silently concentrating on the music, one might actively search for the lyrics to the song, while another will mouth the words while lost in reverie. When testing out this method and slightly increasing the volume for anxiety-filled transition periods, it is important to be mindful of the music we choose. It has to be something familiar and have a certain harmonious ring to it. Something like the Girls' Choir works wonders, at least here in Denmark. But it could just as well be a well-known country song.

*Sensory experiences let us know if a room is safe,
whether we can relax or should be on the alert.*

Lighting

The kind of lighting we choose can make a big difference. We recommend using a variety of light sources and scattering them around the room: on the wall, the ceiling, and on tables. Use different types of lamps and in many different colors. We also use candles (under direct supervision). Combining multiple light sources naturally produces a softer light and gives a soft glow to the room. Where candles are not permitted due to fire regulations, battery-operated candles may be used.

At our home, we use a combination of lights, and many of our lamps are unique antiques or vintage finds. Thus the lighting itself draws upon different periods in the residents' lives and adds authenticity to their surroundings. The flickering light from candles bathes the shared living room in subtle movement and warmth. Two candles on a table are enough to stimulate life and ambiance. When we reach across the table and light a candle, we see the residents let out a sigh of relief. It is just a brief moment, but it seems to give them a sense of peace and calm.

We also have a glass-fronted fireplace at Dagmarsminde. The sight of the flickering flames is compelling, and the residents enjoy sitting and staring into the fire. It provides an intense source of light and heat. A fire in the fireplace, or in our garden firepit, is meditative and draws their attention unlike anything else.

Daylight is equally important. Like everything else, it has to be carefully considered. Many new nursing homes are constructed with enormous windows, bathing the rooms in sunlight—so much that it is almost blinding, which can be disturbing to the residents. For people with dementia, bright sunlight can be uncomfortable. Similarly, light entering the space through skylights can be intense and difficult to control. We let daylight in at particular moments throughout the day, such as when we have said "Good morning" to a resident and pulled up the shades, or when we start the day together at the breakfast table. The residents might note the wind blowing outside and be reminded of the seasons. We are lucky enough to have a view of the sky from many of our windows.

When our residents nap in the afternoon in the resting area connected to the shared living room, we let in a bit of sunlight. If the light gets too sharp or it is too hot, we draw the curtains a little. Falling asleep in sunlight can be like light therapy. Our residents sleep in separate beds in the same room and absorb the light. We believe this sleep–light treatment helps keep depression at bay.

Scent

A nursing home needs to smell clean, but it also needs to smell *good*. Scents—such as rolls baking for breakfast or the cake for coffee in the afternoon—help to create ambience. We all know the wonderful smell of freshly baked bread. It is a happy scent that reminds many of us of our childhood and creates a cozy atmosphere.

At Dagmarsminde, essential oils can help stimulate or lighten the mood. If we want peace and calm, we place drops of lavender into the aroma lamp or diffuser. If the residents need help to relax a little more—and maybe even fall asleep—then notes of cedar can be effective. We might even rub a few drops on our wrists and gently touch the residents' faces; most of the time, an otherwise restless resident will calm down or even go to sleep. When we want to freshen up and invigorate the group, we might choose to use notes of citrus. We usually stay away from grapefruit or orange scents, which can remind people of cleaning agents. We use pure, essential oils, which only require a few drops. Essential oils can also be helpful if a room feels stuffy, which sometimes happens with many people in one room, each exhaling and giving off body heat. In this case, we use cleansing oils developed to freshen the air.

Some locations may have prohibitions against applying essential oils directly on the skin. It is a good idea to research this issue before trying it. Staff in some homes will place a couple of drops on an absorbent surface such as felt, or on a facial tissue placed in the pocket, and thus allow the scent to spread throughout the home as they work.

For us, using scents is a way of showing respect for the people who live at our home. When we drip the oil into the aroma lamp, we are careful to avoid over-scenting the room. This is one of the important daily meaningful little acts of caring.

Dishware

It is equally important to set the table with nicely designed napkins and colorful bouquets. A cup does not have to be an anonymous, white, institutional cup. These mass-produced cups do not inspire residents in any way. Placement of different types of cups in a variety of colors and designs on the table prompts a resident to reach out for a particular cup, hold it, and feel its warmth. In this way, we encourage the resident to use his or her sense of touch and reinforce the ability to drink without assistance.

Textures

Along the same lines, it is important to remember to include some soft items in the living room. Following are examples:

- Lambskins, which are nice to touch
- Beautiful blankets the residents can wrap around themselves when they want to rest or when they get a little chilled sitting still during an activity
- Pillows in a variety of shapes and thicknesses that can be used to support a resident's back or neck or placed under a weak arm

Large and small potted plants give the residents something interesting to look at and attend to. Furs, flowers, and green plants are also a way of inviting nature inside, a kind of meaningful décor, which awakens in our residents an innate feeling of being connected to something greater. Chapter 12 provides more details on the significance of nature.

Tidiness

Clutter creates chaos and confusion in our residents, so we constantly emphasize the importance of staff tidying after themselves. They are in the habit of cleaning up, sanitizing, and throwing out trash at regular intervals. When we end an activity or leave a resident's room, we glance over our shoulder and check:

- Is everything gone, including the glass on the bedtable and the washcloth on the edge of the sink?
- Is there a new bag in the trash can?
- Is the bed made?
- Are the flowers in the vase drooping and in need of removal?

Having an eye for order signals that things are under control. In the residents' state of dependency, they can count on us to maintain a clean and tidy environment.

Gated Garden

We have a big gate at our entrance that is right next to a road with fast-moving traffic. New residents tend to move toward the gate as if they are magnetically drawn to it. When we find them heading in that direction, we walk over and tell them the gate is locked with a code so they cannot leave, and that we do this for their own safety. After a while the residents do not go there anymore; this is partly because of our explanation and partly because we make sure they have more interesting things to do. Gradually, they lose interest or forget about it entirely. Our whole garden is fenced, but—in contrast to what you might think—it actually helps the residents feel free. They can explore every nook and cranny on their own without constant supervision. They can study the plants and stones or gaze out over the fields, undisturbed.

Animals

We discovered early on that pets, such as rabbits, cats, and dogs, can play an important role in our treatment. The pets are sweet and stimulate the resident's sense of touch while offering the comfort of another living being. Everyone, sick or healthy, has an innate need to show affection. I think it is important that animals are an integral part of daily life at the nursing home and not merely used as random entertainment on rare occasions.

We see residents having long conversations with our cat, Herman. Sometimes he will lie in the lap of a resting resident, waiting to be petted and nuzzled when the resident wakes up. The dog gets a pat and a few forbidden treats, and lends support when a person is having difficulty communicating. Residents can sit and quietly pet our rabbits for an hour or so during the day if they want to. It is stimulating and comforting to feel the silky-soft animals.

We also have goats and chickens outside. They live right outside the door, where the residents can watch them as they walk in the garden, feed them by hand, or gather eggs. The little tasks connected to these animals also give the residents a sense of purpose.

Art

The walls at Dagmarsminde are painted white, and we spent a lot of time considering the art we wanted to hang there. We decided to use pictures and paintings of nature, so that residents could immerse themselves in the beautiful pictures and feel a kind of infinity when they contemplate the landscapes. Landscapes are not the only option, of course; it is only important to choose the art carefully and with the interests and cultures of the residents in mind. Art can open up possibilities for a more meaningful experience.

Personal Possessions

The bedroom is the resident's personal space; we always knock before we enter. The room is the person's refuge at night and for short periods throughout the day. We allow our residents to bring some of their personal possessions to our nursing home. For instance, a resident may have picked out a couple of special pieces of furniture with his or her family. In the person's room are pictures on the walls, photo albums, books, and other personally meaningful items chosen by the resident.

Furniture

My overall advice for creating a homey atmosphere is to do what feels natural. Just like any home we have visited or lived in, we want to make our care home a place where we would like to stay. Making a place feel like home does not have to be expensive; in fact, it will never be as expensive as using institutional furniture. I recommend investing in a few unique pieces of furniture for the cozy corners of the living room. A single iconic chair or lamp, thoughtfully designed, can recall memories or initiate conversations between residents. The décor needs to reflect one's goals and ambitions for the room.

The resident's bed is usually placed against the wall in the small but comfortable bedroom. The wall works as a protective border but also gives the resident a good view of the outside. We do everything in our power to avoid hospital beds because they are not normal. A bed is where the resident's day starts and ends, and thus it is an important symbol of security. The person can think, "This is my fortress in the darkness when I am alone in my room at night. Someone will be by my side soon; someone will help me."

The Norm:
A Nursing Home Designed from Fear?

Why do nursing home interiors often give the impression that the residents are a threat to themselves and their surroundings? When I look back at the nursing homes I have worked at or visited, one thing always struck me: Why is the décor so cautious—a what-if-it's-dangerous environment? It seems like backward thinking, considering it is a home where people live. Here are some common features of many nursing homes:

- Chairs upholstered with material that can withstand urine
- Seamless floors, made from something that can stand a lot of dirt and dust
- Slick, laminated tables
- Ceiling lifts in every corner
- Shelves containing posters of books instead of real books
- Pictures dangling from strings attached to the paneling, so they can easily be replaced and sent back

These shared spaces are unsettling; there is a certain transience, a detached coldness to them, as if they could be cleared out at a second's notice. The same goes for the residents' rooms; they are often empty, soulless shells, despite the relatives' ardent attempts to make them cozy. Interiors like these obviously were not designed for normal living. They are designed for people who come with an instruction manual and "bubble wrap." These interiors seem apprehensive of what the residents might do or need. When we let fear be the deciding factor of the décor, we create dysfunctional institutions that make people even sicker.

In 1859, the English nursing icon, Florence Nightingale, wrote that the sick become sicker from always looking at the same wall, the same ceiling, the same surroundings. That was more than 160 years ago, but for many nursing home systems time has apparently stood still. Today's nursing home residents rarely see anything but the same walls—their room or the shared living space—day in and day out.

In addition to this daily monotony, the resident is exposed to a wide spectrum of other unhealthy stimuli, such as bright ceiling lights; empty surfaces; unpleasant smells; replicas on wall posters; poor acoustics; and rigid institutional furniture, like hospital beds, noisy trolleys, and assistive devices with sharp metal edges. These are degrading stimuli, which no one can stand for very long. The whole purpose of a nursing home is to help the residents live well, despite their illness. Instead, we put unnecessary stress on people by placing them in a sick and hollow environment that encourages them to resign to their fate and give up.

Well-Intentioned Dysfunctional Design

Apart from the visibly dysfunctional décor, some nursing homes, despite good intentions, are set up according to fear principles. Below are two classic examples of what I mean.

Camouflaging the halls

Some nursing homes for people with dementia feature doors plastered with images of bookcases, wooden paneling, and so on. This is an attempt to prevent residents who are drawn to the doors from getting out. The idea is to fool the resident so that he or she will stop trying to run away. In some nursing homes, staff even take a picture of the resident's old front door, enlarge it, and stick it on the door to the resident's room, as a way to teach the person how to find the way home.

The bookcases and paneling on the doors only add to the artificiality of the environment. I highly doubt that residents have an easier time finding their own rooms because a picture of their old entrance is glued to their door nor that the residents trying to head outside become less agitated if the exits are camouflaged. We have never used these kinds of strategies at Dagmarsminde, and I can attest to the fact that once residents feel they belong there, they quickly find their way back to the plain white door of their room. If they cannot, we walk them there, and that act alone instills a feeling of belonging and security.

Although staff create these wall-poster devices with the best of intentions, thinking residents will feel safer and be helped by them, these kinds of initiatives often have the opposite effect. They can exacerbate the person's experience of being ill and feeling incompetent, which leads to self-defeat, intensifying the resident's dementia symptoms. The person's self-esteem can drop, and he or she closes off and gets more stressed. Residents may have trouble sleeping, lose their appetite, experience momentary lapses of reality, or become angry and not want to cooperate. The décor becomes an extension of the initial discomfort these residents likely experienced when they first arrived.

Just a job

Many care homes have set up a stereo system, and the whole place is filled with the music, but unfortunately not music chosen with the residents in mind. The staff often just automatically tune in to their own favorite station. In many places, staff do not consider whether the residents are in the mood for classical music, hip-hop, jazz, or classic rock. To make matters worse, carts, walkers, and other assistive devices fill the rooms and hallways—along with the unmistakable stench of urine and stale air.

Most of the relatives I talk with tell me this is what their loved one faces on a daily basis. The staff are lackadaisical because, for them, taking care of people with dementia is "just a job." They do not pay attention to the aesthetics. They claim that the care, not the appearance, is important. However, it is important to fully embrace the personhood of those who live in our homes. They are whole people just as we are. Would you want to live in a home filled with metal furniture, assistive devices, intercoms, and the constant beeping of alarms? Would you enjoy strangers walking through your living room? Of course not; it would make you sick. People with dementia are already having a hard time. We have to think differently about décor from the start.

Objections

"Rugs can be life-threatening."

There are plenty of excuses for not making a care *home* and sticking to an innocuous décor. The logic behind it is often disguised as concern for the resident, but in reality, it is a way of making life easier for the staff, not the resident.

What the statement above (which I've heard numerous times) is actually referring to is that, if a resident is walking around alone at a nursing home without rugs, he or she will be less likely to fall. But why would a resident with dementia be heading somewhere without a staff member in the room? Beyond the fact that a staff member always needs to be present and ready at any moment to guide an unsteady individual, most residents can see when there is a rug on the floor. They also know how to walk across it. Of course, it is always a good idea to choose a heavy rug that will not fold or slide, but the point is, the residents know a rug when they see one. If there is a beautiful rug on the floor, it looks like a well-kept place—a place where people are careful not to spill food, and so on. A neat and tidy place generates neat and tidy behavior. When a home is decorated with rugs and normal furniture, staff are careful and conscientious about what they do. I have found that my staff do not walk across the living room with soiled incontinence pads; they walk around, so as not to soil the carpet.

Residents could trip on a rug; it is a risk. But life is full of risks. The risk that the residents will feel isolated in a dysfunctional environment is even greater. Which risk should inform the design of a home for our elders with dementia?

"This is my workplace, and it should be as safe as possible."

We need to challenge the widespread notion that nursing homes are solely work environments and therefore need to be hazard-free. This view leads to a kind of fearmongering that prevents us from being open to more person-centered approaches to care and can represent a real danger to our residents.

Some may think it is ridiculous to focus on determining the optimal lighting for the shared living room instead of indiscriminately installing fluorescent tubes and cold ceiling lamps because the staff need bright light to work.

But why differentiate between work and home? The staff have nice comfortable lighting at home, so why do they need bright white lights when they are at work? Their vision does not suddenly get worse when they are at work, so the bright lights represent an unnecessary precaution, which I would rather go without. If we need more light to treat a wound or other accident, then we obviously turn on more lights. But when we are talking to each other, making coffee, eating, holding someone's hand, or singing, the bright health and safety lighting is too much.

As mentioned earlier, out of consideration for the residents' safety, many places have done away with candlelight, but once again, if a staff member is on site, which they need to be anyway, they keep an eye on the candles.

"All nursing homes smell bad."

When I say that a nursing home should not smell bad, some respond by saying the smell is to be expected with residents who have urinary incontinence. I disagree. It is the staff's responsibility to prevent accidents and quickly clean them up if they occur. It is also the staff's responsibility to ensure residents do not sit in wet incontinence pads.

Residents who urinate on the floor need to be guided into a routine where they reach the bathroom in time. It is just a matter of organization. I know a pad is supposed to last for 8 hours according to the information on the package, but pads irritate and sting the residents' skin and can lead to fungal or urinary tract infections. Most importantly, though, the residents need to continue to use the bathroom instead of using a pad, just to support their own independence. The nursing home should remain clean and pleasant-smelling.

In response to all the arguments against creating a beautiful and cozy décor, the priority in all these cases should be the resident.

Summary

Whatever décor you end up with, it should feel like *home*. The residents should sense they belong there. Creating a nice, comfortable space for the residents encourages interaction and touch—a squeeze of the shoulder, a hug, holding hands, or the stroke of a cheek.

We need to create completely normal everyday spaces and ensure the residents feel their lives have meaning, so that they will think, *Here I am, and it's a normal place. I'm normal. But I'm also special, because that's what I feel here. I have no second thoughts about being here in this comfortable, nice living room. I know I'm no longer living where I used to, but I live here now—and it's nice.* The environment we are helping to create every day should prioritize the resident's need to live in a home—*their* home—in peace and dignity.

———●◆●———

Questions for Reflection

1. Consider the aesthetic environment of your care home. Which aspects are supportive of a home-like environment, and which are more institutional?

2. Can you imagine some elements of the environment that can be made more cozy? What steps would be involved in making those changes? What, if any, are the obstacles? Try to consider some strategies for addressing them.

3. Which aspects of the aesthetics as described at Dagmarsminde would be more, or less, helpful to the people in your care?

3

The Craft of Nursing

Good Judgment and Hands-on Care

GOOD JUDGMENT IS ESSENTIAL FOR creating a caring care home. Therefore, it is crucial that good judgment is nurtured and celebrated, and why it is one of the main virtues I focus on in this chapter. Another virtue that deserves recognition is touch, the work we do with our hands. Both judgment and touch represent a return to the core values of nursing.

Learning the Craft of Nursing

When I was 17 and in my final years at secondary school, I got a job at a local state-run nursing home. It was my first encounter with care work. I enjoyed being at the nursing home and quickly understood how much I could learn by spending time with the older residents. I learned to decode their language. They did not always speak with words but with sounds or body language, and I was driven to understand their communication.

I also learned a lot from my colleagues. Some of the older nurses became my greatest role models. In particular, Rita taught me some of the fundamental skills of nursing, which I still use today. Rita always told me to "see how the land lies" before entering a resident's room. Most of the nurses would just burst in when they had to attend to something. Rita always quietly knocked, waited, and calmly entered, assessing the mood before she spoke or attended to the resident.

Among those Rita cared for was a woman with dementia, who was often very aggressive. We quickly had to interpret and figure out the meaning of her expressions—what she needed— or she would get furious. Rita knew how, and she had developed a good rapport with this resident. The woman was not just complicated to work with; her actions toward others could be outright harmful. For instance, she called one nurse ugly and told her that her mother must have regretted giving birth to her. She would react with this type of cutting expression when we did not set her glass on her preferred corner of the table or return her hearing aid to exactly the right place inside the case on the nightstand. When we helped her put on her nightgown, she demanded we pull the fabric down tight to mid-thigh, and we had to stretch it like a bedsheet to reach; if we pulled it an inch farther she would strike at us like a snake. The day she died my other colleagues were relieved, but not Rita. She had befriended the resident, and so had I.

Good Judgment

My experience with Rita taught me about one of the most important tools we use as caregivers, namely, good judgment. Guidelines for dementia care are often on display in the staff room at nursing homes or taught in courses. But the wonderful thing about developing our own judgment is that we do not have to get stuck in pre-set ideas. Our judgment is an inherent, intuitive sense directing our every move in a specific care situation or for the specific person we are caring for. It is the ability to perceive, to make up our mind, and to engage.

The entire care sector is so saturated with instruments, evidence, technological aids, medicine, protocols, rules, and procedures that many of us have forgotten to tune in to our own gut feeling. It seems like light-years since anyone last highlighted the fact that nursing is essentially a craft. We have to keep asking ourselves, "What do I perceive and believe, and how does that influence my work with the vulnerable individual who now needs my care?"

At Dagmarsminde, our good judgment also influences our ability to be creative and to empathize. When we choose care as a treatment form, we have to scrap the conventional guidelines. Without any pre-set care models (clinical diagnosis terminology), we can start by using our own discretion. But we have to believe in our process. We have to trust each individual staff member's judgment skills, allowing him or her to draw from personal experience and intuition—what comes from living life, training as a nurse, hearing advice from colleagues and relatives—and also from the staff member's own doubt, which must be noticed and attended to.

Life at Our Home

I once went to help a woman in one of the rooms at Dagmarsminde. Her short-term memory had completely deteriorated. Yet she was still perfectly capable of getting up in the morning, taking a shower, and so on. We had to be somewhere nearby, passing in and out of her room, but giving her the space to take care of things herself. One morning I was serving coffee for some residents in the living room, and everything seemed normal—other than my gut feeling that something was not right, and it really bothered me. I could not figure out what was going on. I sensed I needed to check on the resident to see if she was on her way to join us. It was earlier than her usual wakeup time, and I knew she would be irritated and stressed if I interrupted her in the bathroom. But when I knocked and opened the door, I witnessed a strange scene. There were clothes everywhere, and the woman was pacing the room in her underwear, complaining she could not find her clothes, while trying to tidy at the same time. She had broken out in a cold sweat and was deeply frustrated. She said she was so embarrassed and that she was a stupid old lady. I didn't know what to do. Should I sit her down on the bed and talk to her? Hold her?

My decision was based on what I'd sensed entering the room. I quietly led her into the bathroom and said, "You were about to take a shower, right? I'll get the water running while you get undressed." She got under the showerhead, and when I was sure she was actually washing herself, I went out of the bathroom but left the door slightly ajar. Then I cleaned up the room, putting most of the clothes back in the closet and a little pile in the laundry basket. I made her bed, but also cleaned off her little table, which she had covered with shreds of toilet paper. As soon as I heard her fiddling with the showerhead to turn it off, I was back by her side again. When we came out of the bathroom, she was tired, but looked around and said, "Oh, I've already cleaned up. I guess I'm ready then."

When we consistently work on our judgment skills, we realize this work goes hand-in-hand with doubt, which often increases as our judgment improves. It is only natural that we should be uncertain about the situations we face. The important thing is to remember to be open about that doubt: What is it trying to tell us about this particular situation, and how can we learn to use doubt as a tool and as a basis for further developing our judgment skills?

Working at Full Throttle—Slowly

There is no template for good judgment, but give it some space and it can be powerful. Alongside judgment, we try to take an approach I call "working at full throttle—slowly." What do I mean by that? I am not talking about rushing from one task to another; I am talking about seeing the work as something more than an endless series of tasks.

For example, a resident may be showing signs of frustration and having a hard time dealing with his anger. When we are busy and need to tend to the next resident, we might think to ourselves, "He's always mad. Typical 'frontal lobe damage.'" Instead, when we work at full throttle—slowly, we can find the time to figure out what is bothering the person. We could sit down and talk with him about it, and we could acknowledge his frustration, saying, "I can't believe it," and so on. Or maybe we could quietly approach him, make eye contact, and speak to him in a low voice. We hold back a little. These situations can be hard work as we fine tune our senses and decide how to tackle the problem. When the resident has our acknowledgment, he feels seen and understood, and he will usually calm down. In this case, we were able to rein in his frustration, but in the meantime our mind may have churned a million miles a minute with doubts about our ability to handle the situation. We had our doubts, mustered up the courage, decided on something, and signaled our compassion and acceptance.

> When a resident has our acknowledgment, he feels seen and understood, and he will usually calm down.

Another example of working slowly at full throttle is when a resident is having trouble feeding herself. The other residents around the table find her eating issues disgusting. They get irritated and openly declare that they do not want to sit next to her. If we remove the resident for the sake of the others,

Life at Our Home

One of our residents could not speak and was in a difficult phase of her Parkinson's disease. She would suddenly burst into tears and we did not know why. We tried one gentle approach after another: Was it the light? Too much noise? Was she sitting wrong in her chair? We tried everything—massage, having her lie down for a while, and so forth. Nothing stopped the sudden outbursts. Then one of the staff members gave her a glass of juice with a short straw and she immediately stopped crying. I asked my colleague how she thought of it. She could not explain why, but it almost always worked. Ever since then, we have had a glass of water or juice with a short straw close at hand. It's not that she was thirsty, but that the straw provided a kind of oral stimulation and focus, which got her to stop crying.

she will feel excluded. Instead, by involving everyone around the table, by expressing empathy and helping the resident wipe her mouth, by speaking affectionately to her, and by creating an awareness of her situation—maybe even telling the angry resident across from her that the resident needs his help too, so she can get enough to eat—we generate a shared concern for the individual at the table, even if we have to do the same thing again the very next day.

Within our little community at Dagmarsminde, we often see residents empathizing with other residents who have difficulties. Sometimes they even step in and lend a hand. They want to show affection. It is important that we include everyone, even the resident who was having trouble eating. This can be challenging; it means staying focused and engaging at the same time. This is what I mean by working at full throttle—slowly. Working with this mindset, we find that a simple solution is often the best.

The Value of Touch

Another one of the core values of the Dagmarsminde approach is using our hands. It might sound strange to even mention it, but using one's hands and, even more importantly, talking about it in the process, emphasizing it, is an essential part of our care treatment; it is the tactile element of nursing. When we touch another human being and acknowledge the energy between us, we gain insight into the care that is needed. It creates a connection between the staff member and the resident, both on an inner and an outer level, revealing the resident's needs and better enabling the staff member to fulfill them.

Holding a resident's hand is an intimate moment and can confirm or dismiss the person's need for affection. He or she might pull back the hand, which tells the staff member a boundary has been overstepped. The resident might not yet share the trust assumed by the staff member. When we decide whether or not a resident is ready for us to enter his or her personal space, we have to gauge the person's openness to us and to the help we offer. We cannot just decide on our own how a resident needs to be helped.

Caring for a resident should be a harmonious process. If the resident reaches out to us, it is a sign he or she needs something. The person might have something specific to tell us, but often residents just need to ascertain that we are there and are looking out for them. It is then the staff member's responsibility not to see holding the person's hand as the solution, but to consider what the request really means, to find out what the resident is trying to communicate by physically reaching out.

We deliberately use touch to give residents a feeling of closeness and comfort, for example when we hold a restless resident's shoulders or grip the ankles of someone lying down to rest. There are different ways to touch, but the general rule is that the energy a staff member transfers to the resident needs to be encouraging and light. How can we tell, you may ask. We can feel it. We transfer our loving thoughts for the resident's condition through our hands. The resident usually calms down, breathes a little easier, smiles, or even opens up and tells the staff member something important.

Massage is a form of touch. We have a massage therapist who visits every other week and gives the residents a massage suited to their individual needs. But that is not enough, so the staff also give massages and other kinds of meaningful touch. We constantly use our hands, for everything from rubbing sensitive areas with moisturizing cream to helping residents sleep. Our staff members are not all trained in massage, but they try different techniques and learn by doing. For example, we like to use massage as a part of the morning ritual when the residents are still in bed. It warms their skin and energizes them. Their joints and muscles relax and they have an easier time edging their way out of bed and onto their feet. Waking up to this kind of touch helps the person feel up to getting out of bed and up to tackling life.

We also use our hands to prevent acute conditions—both mental and physical—through conscious touch. We can touch a resident's skin and feel if he or she has a fever, swelling, or any sore areas. We can also use touch to sense any forthcoming agitation. A resident's skin will feel cold and moist, and the pulse will be racing. Then we know we have to act quickly to prevent any self-destructive behavior. Caring for people with dementia means constantly anticipating each resident's needs and fulfilling them before it is too late. By using our hands, we strive to improve a resident's connection to his or her own body.

Our core values—good judgment and using our hands—encourage care partners to be in touch with their senses, including not just seeing, but also listening to the nuances of a resident's sounds. Consider the tone of a resident's voice. Is it too high or does it sound a little heavy? These are signs of a resident's mood. Our methods are founded on traditional nursing values, in which the staff member's body is always interacting with the resident. We believe in the original, natural methods, which offer residents a harmonious life so they can relate to—and become an integral part of—what we do.

The Norm: Another Day at the Care Home "Factory"

Employees at nursing homes are often encouraged to view the work they do as just that, work. Instead of the well-being of residents in their care being the central focus, the goal of nursing as work can become the ticked box, the completed form, or the accomplished tasks. How do we ensure we are not encouraging an environment based on attaining goals more suited to productivity targets for staff working on shifts at a factory?

Tasks, Rather Than Care?

In many nursing homes, a workday starts when the staff member enters a resident's room. At the top of the checklist is, "Clean private parts of bedridden resident." The checklist also notes that this resident needs pureed or softened (swallow-friendly) food. The wording might seem tactful and professional, even positively framed, but absent is a sense of the whole person and the helpfulness of the tasks for him or her. The dutiful staff member gets started on the daily tasks—one by one—until the end of his or her shift. Care work today is often structured around procedures to improve workflow and efficiency. The productivity of the individual care worker is constantly being measured.

The same routine repeats day after day. The tasks may be completed, but if residents have been resistant or have not been able to comply with the completion of these tasks, they will not be getting the help they need. The resistance may be explained as just another irreversible symptom of the disease, a part of dementia, and therefore the outcome has been as good as could be expected—and another box checked.

Thus, the machine keeps churning. When the focus is on tasks first rather than care first, people drawn to care work find themselves up against productivity metrics to stay employed; those in their care suffer when the time required to nurture human connection is not valued.

Fun-Filled Activities, for Whom?

Offering a schedule of activities is often another box to tick, another goal to accomplish. The staff of the care factory, in their efforts to provide "fun-filled activity," might arrange a little entertainment for the residents. They believe they are doing something special for their residents. But in these efforts to provide things to do, the nursing home can miss providing choices that are meaningful and interesting for its residents.

It is also important to be sure the activities are part of what any of us as older adults might enjoy. Activities that make us laugh and bring joy are good, but they should remain age appropriate, setting appropriate, and respectful. I am going to share what I hope is an extreme example to make this point. I once saw a program on TV about a nursing home and a special approach the staff had to entertaining their residents. They lined them up in the hallway and gave them each a carrot because they were bringing a pony up the elevator to the third floor. The staff were all smiles and thought it was hilarious. The residents looked happy, and the viewers probably were too. A clip shared on social media about the pony visit went viral. It was a funny film, but at whose expense? It's easy to laugh. But a pony in a living room is not normal. And bewildered residents holding carrots does not send a message to viewers that these members of our society are valued and worthy of respect. Think of the time the staff put into planning this event to ensure their residents a good time.

In fairness, the pony visit was probably orchestrated with the best intentions. Sometimes these kinds of events are successful and fun for the residents. But this way of thinking eludes the central question: Is there any value in it for the residents? Is it making them feel safe in their own home, or is it just weird? I believe the choice of something weird probably reflects how the planners see the residents—as weird.

It is hard to tell from the viral video if the staff had discussed beforehand what leading a pony down the hall might mean for the residents. Looking at it from a professional standpoint might have led the staff to question whether the initiative was in line with the care home's core values of inclusion and meeting the individuals' needs. I am also certain that most of the residents would say ponies do not belong inside.

It is important to remember that most people with dementia, despite the disease, still have a clear notion of what is normal or not. To understand, we have to return to the residents' perception of their own lives. Many would tell us they feel healthy and normal but that they are living in a reality that seems abnormal, sometimes bordering on the absurd.

There is no point in parading ponies inside a nursing home or arranging other shows that are silly for the setting. These sorts of events are not beneficial for the people living there. There are so many meaningful initiatives to plan instead. A picnic in the forest, yoga in the garden, a live concert in the living room, an evening around the firepit—these are all activities

that belong to the real world, the world the residents live in and
know. At Dagmarsminde, our goal is to offer our residents a life
filled with contentment, love, and respect.

Technological Wonders, or Are They?

Technological wonders invented to help with dementia belong
in the same category as ill-considered activity initiatives. Such
inventions may have been developed with good intentions, but
when their implementation substitutes for human connection,
the craft of care we want to practice is lost and the residents do
not benefit. Here are a few examples:

- High-definition wide-screen TVs with nature scenes or
  other programming meant to engage residents with "stimulating" pictures. Residents often sit in front of these, but
  ignore them.

- Massage chairs, or so-called sensory chairs. For example, the enormous bean bag with large heavy flaps that
  wrap around a resident like a big hug can offer a sense of
  safety and security but may just leave the resident feeling
  isolated.

- Robotic plush animals or dolls. Purchased on the assumption that they will help residents feel calm and happy,
  these devices are too often age inappropriate or confusing.

The staff may benefit from these "wonders" if time spent finding ways to generate comfort and joy for residents is reduced,
but the results for residents likely are not the outcomes the caring nursing home really wants. Inanimate objects and software
should not substitute for the personal engagement and sensory
experiences residents deserve.

For me, these kinds of care devices convey a sense of professional resignation, a loss of our goals for good care. Their use
may be a red flag, signaling that the leaders of the care home
value technological substitutions over creating a setting that
supports staff in making real connections with residents. As
an example, when a resident becomes increasingly disruptive,

restlessly wandering up and down the halls, a scramble ensues to find any solution to pacify the person. The default at the care factory is frequently to turn to technology instead of devoting staff time. But does investing large sums of money in activities and technology truly enhance caring?

We do not have any mechanical pets at Dagmarsminde, nor do we want any. Robotic pets do not compensate for the human touch and comfort we provide, and we don't need the added expenditures in our budget. Care technology does not help residents feel grounded or give them a sense of belonging. Taking people outside to feel the air on their faces, to touch a tree, or to help water the flowers will also be a better way to appreciate nature than to look at a picture of a forest on a big screen. This is the type of sensory experience to foster. The use of devices, instead of helping, can lead to semi-comatose, under-stimulated elders. Care staff end up distancing themselves from the human they wanted to reach. What then? The residents only get more debilitated, and possibly sick—increasing the risk of hospitalization.

Ironically, we often face the same issue with children. Parents are repeatedly warned against leaving their children with the iPad or in front of the TV. There is a pervasive, justified worry about the consequences of their spending too much time in front of a screen. We need to have the same concerns for the older adults in our care.

Objection:
"We're doing everything we can . . ."

Are we practicing our craft of care when people who cannot speak or move sit for hours in a corner in a wheelchair or a bean bag? Are we practicing our craft of care if someone sits in a wet incontinence pad? Are we practicing our craft of care if we think it will not hurt to surf the internet while "feeding dinner" to a person with dementia? Are we practicing our craft of care if we do not try our hardest to understand the communication of someone with Parkinson's disease?

Maybe a furrowed brow is a call for help. To say, without a second thought, "That resident can't speak," is neglect. Are we practicing our craft of care when we do not try to figure out what the 77-year-old woman is telling us with her constant, loud hello, and we wave it off as "just her thing"? Are we practicing our craft of care if we prioritize coffee breaks and shift-handoff meetings over being together with the residents? No, we are not.

We can avoid leaving residents who have lost the ability to speak sitting alone and staring. When leadership and staff members use their intuition and their good judgment, they learn to decode what the residents are trying to communicate. Is that leg that keeps twitching actually a sign of discomfort?

If the residents do not sense any response, they will begin to withdraw from the outside world. They give up. They must not be moved into a corner and forgotten. That is a terrible neglect.

Summary

Our public health care sector, once founded on principles of empathy and good judgment, has become focused on science-driven solutions, where approaches to disease revolve around chemical and technological innovations. Only solutions that can be proven—through numbers or results—are recognized. This is often referred to as evidence-based care work. The healthcare industry is saturated with exclusively evidence-based thinking that can put the craft of caring at peril.

Instead of letting the virtues and knowledge from the past slip into oblivion, we can put them to use again and provide the kind of care in which our senses interact with the patient, the kind that existed for hundreds of years before everything became so science based. It is a good thing we now have antibiotics, anesthetics, medical instruments and equipment, and so much more. But we should not abandon the methods and tools that have existed for millennia, which nurses and other care workers have always known were effective against certain illnesses and imbalances: our good, professional judgment and our hands.

———•◆•———

Questions for Reflection

1. Have you been inspired by the approach of someone who trained you or with whom you work? List some aspects of their care approach that inspire you.

2. Are there tasks in nursing care that seem like "checking boxes" without a real focus on the person you are caring for? Can you think of a way to bring a more person-centered approach to tasks needing to be done?

3. Is there an idea or concept in this chapter that particularly resonates with you? Describe it in your own words and see how it could relate to your own care work.

4

The Call to Service

The Selfless Workplace

IN ADDITION TO THE CRAFT of nursing, the call to service is fundamental to staffing the kind of nursing home I want to see. At Dagmarsminde, our aim is a selfless workplace with free-thinking staff. That does not mean staff members act on their whims. It means they are encouraged to think independently and to let go of many of the methods and templates they have been accustomed to.

Building something from the bottom up takes time for any organization; the same is true for leaders who are trying to implement changes in their approach to care. In the beginning, it is important to establish the values and the view of humanity behind the approach. These should be apparent in every aspect of the organization. Therefore, this call to service is inextricably linked with good leadership. It requires a strong director, who will lead the group and maintain the core values. Staff members who do not agree with these values—sometimes even directly contradicting them—do not belong on the team.

Building a Team

When I founded Dagmarsminde, it took me at least half a year to build my team. Along the way, I had to dismiss several people who were not on the same path as I was. That probably sounds harsh, but it is necessary to carry out the vision. Also, once people are in place, it is important to stay alert to any needed changes. I am constantly refining my team.

How can we choose staff who are naturally suited for the job? We usually choose from among a broad spectrum of applicants for our open positions. Some are from traditional nursing homes and wholeheartedly believe in that system. Others are looking for a new challenge; they are tired of working in the standardized care home sector and have the courage to do something different.

Reinforcing the core values of an existing nursing home also means re-evaluating whether current staff members are qualified for the job. We have to remain focused on our goals and see for ourselves whether staff listen, understand, and carry forward the values of the organization in their interactions with the residents. The goal is to retain loyal staff who will inherently represent the fundamental values of a place.

When I hire new staff, I first look for the right credentials. If we are hiring a new nurse, the applicant must have a degree in nursing. Beyond that, I put away the CV or resume. I would rather see the person sitting in front of me. Is he or she making eye contact? Do I feel good in the person's company? Do the applicant's eyes light up when talking about our care home? Do I have an easy time talking, and laughing, with him or her? Does the person immediately understand what we are doing in this place? What do they feel they can contribute? If an applicant tells me they there are applying here because they "live nearby," that is a red flag for me. I am looking for employees who have something special to offer—something greater than a short drive to and from work.

I appreciate when applicants share what they would like to do or put forward ideas that would suit our care home, which may not have been welcome at the other places they worked. For example, if someone says, "I like knitting, and I would enjoy doing that with the residents," it tells me something about that person's view of humanity; he or she truly wants to engage with the residents. In contrast, it is very telling if the applicant kicks off the interview by asking about "additional vacation days," for instance.

Sometimes I have had an urgent need to fill a specific role and was therefore forced to hire too quickly. It usually does not work out. When possible, I recommend being patient and allowing time for a more considered hiring process. I have found it always to be worth the effort.

The New Employee

We ordinarily do not have a long training period here at Dagmarsminde. The new staff member is a part of the team from the start, and we gradually increase his or her responsibilities. If our new colleague seems to settle in from day one, we know we have made the right choice. Settling in means having a natural inclination to converse with the residents on an equal footing and relate to them easily—thus enabling the new employee to be able to assess the needs of the people in his or her care.

Some new staff members naturally step forward as responsible, hard-working, and eager representatives of our core values. They quickly come up with new initiatives that fall in line with our shared goals. They are our "visionary flag bearers." This is not an official title, but it quickly becomes clear that these individuals genuinely believe in the bigger picture and can serve as an inspiration to both existing and newer colleagues. In some organizations, this kind of enthusiasm gets rebuked by gossip, undermined, and quietly sabotaged—this can happen when a leader is trying to steer a group of individuals toward a common goal. When I first opened Dagmarsminde, only a few of my staff were visionary flag bearers. But when I look at my team now, at least half of my staff seem to have taken on the role. It is not always those who have been here for a while. I often see new staff members pick up the banner from day one. The fresh enthusiasm they bring is essential for the team.

Importance of Leadership

It is helpful for the leader to maintain a constant dialogue with the staff about the overall vision and core values, both in passing remarks and in scheduled meetings and conversation. Always listen to and engage the staff, giving them room to speak, and even letting them speak first. Leadership is not about being tyrannical—it is often just checking that everyone is working in the same direction and from the same values. Of course, most importantly, the director needs to fully believe in and adhere to the home's vision.

Recognition of Good Work

In the standard care world, employees gain recognition by doing things that are not directly connected to the patients or the residents. For example, the staff might expect special acknowledgment for swapping their hours, making a cake for their colleagues, urging a fellow staff member not to strain themselves, registering information in the journals, or completing basic task plans. Also, they receive special praise for helping a resident put on a nice shirt, taking a walk with residents, or singing to them. These kinds of tasks are expected—not extra—at our care home.

At Dagmarsminde, we acknowledge everything that directly improves our residents' lives. That means we only praise an employee for doing something for their colleagues if it means someone will have more time with the residents. For example, if the members of the night watch team prepare more than they need to, or if the daytime workers put in an extra effort sorting out details, the next team can give more attention to the residents. This kind of consideration—ultimately with the residents in mind—is praiseworthy in our book.

Many traditional nursing homes recognize staff workers for doing basic everyday tasks that are expected of them, whereas we praise people for going above and beyond the call of duty. Employees who get credit for doing what is expected of them lower their ambitions and may not be motivated to go out of their way.

Here are a few examples of care for which we reserve special praise:

- Giving a facial to a resident who is restless and unable to sleep
- Preparing a colorful drink with a straw and a little umbrella for a resident, thereby preventing an anxious situation
- Decorating a resident's room before a visit from a relative whose birthday it is, and finding a little gift the resident—who does not remember the visitor's birthday—can give

There will always be some people who are more difficult to lead than others. Some are able to change their mindset, whereas others will have to seek opportunity elsewhere, within a system that suits them. What is important is that all staff understand and believe in what we are trying to do. We can disagree on how to solve a problem; a difference in opinion can be healthy. But a director should always listen and, at the same time, be attuned to whether a dispute is actually a difference in opinion about core values.

For instance, one of our core values at Dagmarsminde is that all residents eat together in the main living space. There is no point in arguing about that and suggesting the residents eat in their rooms; it goes against what we believe. Another core value is that we never give the residents sedatives. So there is no use in suggesting we try sedatives. Other organizations may do things differently and operate on a different set of values. At Dagmarsminde, we hold to the values that we have found to be beneficial for our residents.

Staff Independence

When I say our staff are "independent," I mean that the individual staff member is free to navigate on his or her own within our system of values. Everyone is fully aware of our shared purpose and the empathetic approach that will help us fulfill that purpose. Reaching that point with our team allows us to loosen the reins a little. Staff members have different ways of working together as a team on different shifts. I never get involved in that. They have their own dynamic and enjoy the freedom that comes with working in their own way.

My staff often propose different creative initiatives for how best to complete a task. I discuss it with them and approve it, usually in the presence of other staff members. It is important to broadcast when someone has done something brilliant or innovative to improve a resident's quality of life. This is what I mean by "a selfless workplace"—acknowledging each other for the good of the resident. It is not about highlighting oneself, but about listening and rising together.

A leader has to be both player and coach, being present and following along with what is going on. We have to be inspirational on a higher, philosophical, and value-based level, but the staff also inspire us through their actions and solutions to everyday issues. In this way, ideology and practice are woven together. Employees need to be able to seek out the director if they have doubts about something, and we have to understand that the things we try do not always work out as well as we thought they would. The staff need to be free to be creative and not afraid to raise an issue when a problem arises.

Life at Our Home

At one point we had a resident who did not want to eat. She was nearing the final phase of her illness and no longer understood that she needed to put food in her mouth and chew. A staff member sat down behind the resident, gently holding her forehead while she tried to feed her, and the resident ate. It was the very opposite of what we have been taught—that we need to sit in front of the individual and be a mirror image. This staff member used "180-degree thinking" in this case, and it worked!

Life at Our Home

Once, we were trying to help a younger resident improve her ability to walk. Ordinarily we make a rule of always praising a resident when he or she accomplishes something or achieves a goal. Our praise, however, seemed to have the opposite effect on this resident. Every time we acknowledged her hard work after a training session, or very carefully went through the different methods we used, she withdrew. I realized that none of it made sense to her. Because she did not believe she had a medical condition, she could not understand why she needed to do the exercises. She had no reason to reach any goals; as far as she was concerned, she was fine as she was. Once we realized that, we began to act as if nothing special was happening when she achieved a goal. We would walk with her but not praise her for that, thus not reminding her of her own declining abilities. Her walking improved once we removed the focus from her legs. We ordinarily communicate everything we do with the residents so they understand and are motivated by it. But for this resident, it felt like a direct confrontation with her illness. So we broke with our own system. This is an example of how we are constantly developing and adjusting our approaches in the interest of benefiting the residents.

The Selfless Workplace

When I talk about the call to service at the selfless workplace, I am referring to our inherent need to care for one another, just as we care for our residents. It is a fundamental human need, which we are born with—to be there for another, as the other is there for you. If this natural instinct toward other people is transferred to our work at a care home, we will naturally think of the resident's needs first and try to fulfill them without expecting anything in return. We will not be expecting to be seen or praised, or to know we are doing the right thing, going to Heaven, and so on. That kind of thinking does not lead to *caring* care work.

When we are helping a resident out of bed, our first concern should not be the difficulty of the work: "This is too heavy for me. I had better get a lift." Instead, we think: "Let me see if I can help the resident out of bed some other way." When we show the resident that we believe he or she can get up with a little support—if one or two people are able to lend a hand and physically help the person—it generally works out. On the other hand, if the resident senses hesitancy in us, we are signaling that we do not trust his or her ability and that one of us might be injured. The staff worker's anxiety can make the resident feel responsible for the accident that has not happened yet. Sometimes, we do have to resort to assistive devices, but only after we have determined that it is impossible to lift the person without mechanical help. We do not want to encourage residents to lose faith or confidence in themselves. If we stay focused on helping residents to help themselves, it is better for them.

Sometimes I ask staff members, "Who are you worried about right now?" The question serves as a reminder that, first and foremost, we are here to help the residents. Residents always come first. I realize this is a somewhat rigid stance, but there is good reason for this. When our whole mind is set toward benefiting the resident, we find that residents are more willing to participate. In the end, that makes our job a little easier. There are of course also times when, after numerous attempts, we have to take command and get the resident going by being a kind of compassionate authoritarian. But we use that approach only after *numerous* attempts. Usually, when residents see that we are working for their benefit, they tend to participate actively in their own care.

First and foremost, we are here to help the residents.

Taking a Break

In many care homes I have visited, the staff members start off the day by taking a break. They meet in the morning, sit down with their colleagues, and enjoy a cup of coffee or a fresh roll.

Thus, the first hour of the day quickly passes. For scheduled breaks throughout the day, the staff sit in a room cut off from the residents. The day is planned around these break times. This approach does not lead to a change in the culture of care.

The employee who says, "I need a break," is asking for a break from the residents. I realize that once in a while the residents can be intense. But for us, breaks are not an option; taking breaks from the residents would allow us to escape the very reason we are here. On the whole, independent staff members do not need those kinds of breaks. Instead, it should feel gratifying to be with the residents. They say and do so many inspiring things, and help us to grow as human beings.

I am opposed to taking breaks from the ones we are here to care for. On the other hand, I very much support having the time and space for reflection and contemplation. We make time for reflection—a brief moment of calm and quiet with the residents or a short interlude with a colleague to chat about work. But the focal point should always be the residents.

It is important to remember that we are often seated when we are working, doing things with the residents, trying to put them at ease. It is possible to sit at the shared dining table and hold a resident's hand while also enjoying a cup of coffee in the

Life at Our Home

While I was writing these pages, I took a break to eat lunch with the staff and residents in our shared living space. The sun shone through the windows, and as the group was quiet, I said: "It's so nice and sunny in here." The woman across from me lit up with a smile and said, "It's warming my back." I was deeply touched by her words; it was a perfectly genuine response. I did not think twice about the fact that her mouth was full of food. It was a shared moment between two people, which I would not have experienced sitting in the staff room talking with colleagues.

other hand. When our residents rest after lunch, the employees have some time to themselves. This is when they prepare the rest of the day's activities and discuss the residents' well-being with other staff members.

I usually tell my new colleagues: "Keep in mind, there are no breaks here. But on the other hand, it's a nice place to work, and you get a lot in return. It's intense. When you go home, you're done for the day, and you are probably also tired. But that's what it takes when we go the distance for the residents."

Working with the Call

Some people assume that when I talk about bringing back the call to nursing, it has something to do with getting paid properly. That is not the point here. The staff are salaried, allotted vacation, and receive a pension. But once these terms are set, we enter a world in which work is about what happens between the residents and us, and we are fully engaged with those in our care and with our profession. It makes me happy to see how inspired and independent our employees become. The space is filled with their energy, which is reflected in the tone of their voices and the momentum of our discussions. A conversation about work conditions and pay rates is not nearly as satisfying.

Working from the point of view of the call offers so many positive experiences. With this approach, we see new possibilities open up. Residents who had been unable to talk or move can suddenly speak in full sentences, express joy, and maybe even take a few steps again. It is gratifying to glimpse feelings of normality and confidence in our residents. Staff share these experiences with each other, which helps to keep us all motivated. We enjoy a kind of healthy competition, each of us working in our own way to achieve new heights with the residents. We celebrate our successes together, and staff discover strengths and abilities they may not have known they had. While this approach benefits the staff, it is also helpful for the residents.

The Norm:
Where Is the Call?

Breakthrough change is rare in nursing homes here in Denmark as well as throughout the world. Given the wide variety of models for running and financing care for older adults with dementia, this book focuses primarily on what happens within the nursing home, no matter where it is. And that begins with leadership.

The Director

To start, let's look at the most obvious signs that someone is *not* a good leader—and what that means for daily life at nursing homes. First, many directors of nursing homes do not participate in the direct care of residents. Leaders like these are almost literally invisible because they are always behind a desk—often in a distant corner of the care home. Their work schedule mainly consists of "important" meetings and calling in substitute staff when people call out sick.

Many directors will pull the staff aside and "instruct" them because this kind of behavior is expected in their position, and they can check some kind of professional box for doing so. However, the person may be clueless as to what the staff are in fact doing on the floors because his or her position does not require visiting the floors. Sometimes, one of these leaders may say he or she is listening, but with a false sense of empathy: "I hear what you're saying . . ." This person may hear the employee's words but will not try to understand what is actually at stake for the individual. A director of an organization can never gain any real insight without physically showing up and being present where the work is being done.

Nursing home systems or locations looking for a new director can sometimes get it wrong from the start: the job description. The prospective director must have a degree in administration and must be a well-known professional in the field. In these cases, hiring is based on a confusing set of values created by the current trends for care work. An incompetent director can easily rattle off the system's core values, which have been printed and filed accordingly, and is swelling with empty platitudes about "being there for the individual" and "adapting care to individual needs," and appreciating a work culture that operates "like family." But no one ever assesses whether the director actually lives up to those care objectives—least of all the residents and their families.

Many directors of nursing homes were once employees who are no longer passionate about the work. They may have gone back to school and completed a higher degree, which qualifies them for an administrative or leadership position. Be cautious, however, about the hazards of this career trajectory. A degree in management can be a way of escaping the physical and emotional work of care. Either by choice or as a result of shifting responsibilities, leaders often find themselves sitting in an office, ensuring protocols are maintained, setting schedules and procedures, and performing other administrative functions that do not involve interacting with the residents and staff. This disconnect can give rise to incompetence and low morale among all staff, which of course will have an effect on the residents in their care.

Incompetent leaders are not very demanding, and they do not support growth and improvement in their staff. An incompetent leader may require that all rules and procedures be followed to the letter, but then staff are not encouraged to find effective, creative solutions to unexpected problems that arise in the lives of their residents. When everyone follows a set model, it may look good "on paper," but residents do not benefit from this approach. When journalists report that residents sit alone in their rooms looking dirty and unkempt, that the staff members are known to run private errands during their shift, that a resident has died because of neglect, or that the staff sick leave has increased to 5 weeks a year, the system may fire the incompetent director to avert the public scrutiny. Perhaps it will help to have a new leader, but if the system leadership was happy with the status quo until it became known publicly, it is unlikely that just changing administrators will shift the culture of care in that system. Often, the new administrator begins with promises to do better, and over time nothing changes.

Effect of Poor Leadership on Staff and Residents

After a while, poor leadership starts affecting the morale of the employees. They walk around confused, without direction. Naturally, they start counting the days before their vacation and counting the minutes before their next break for coffee, cake, or a cigarette.

When I present lectures to people who work in the care sector, I sometimes meet a tired, inattentive crew, whose eyes are glazed over or are absorbed by their phones or the doodlings in their notebooks. As employees, they have switched off. Once people reach that point of indifference, there is no end to the issues that can arise. Some staff become defiant. Without guidance and reinforcement of core values, an organization can become rife with people wanting to change processes according to their own preferences or even lead others in that direction. Someone may decide not to go along with one or more of the daily procedures for waking residents, serving meals, leading activities, or any of the smaller customs and practices, such as whether or not to light candles. One person might say to a colleague, "Why don't you take the rest of the day off?" (In other words: "So will I.") Someone with a different work ethic may make up excuses for not working with the residents, supposedly in the name of safety. "Be careful of your back. You might hurt yourself." (In other words: "Don't work too hard. You'll make the rest of us look bad.")

Another might exaggerate the need to avoid a resident: "Look out for that guy, he's a little unpredictable and violent. Don't get too close to him." Different employees have different perspectives on what is wrong, but their reports often focus on everything other than the well-being of the residents. This disunity of purpose makes the care home a sad place to be, where the residents are mostly just in the way, and where the only thing you might hear in the empty foyer is the static from the sports channel.

This is a place that is both stalling and full of people who each want the home to operate according to their own values, and there is no real leader. People become enemies and group together, and daily life at the care home is more about staff problems than the challenges faced by the residents. Because of low morale and low staffing, nursing homes often attempt to fill the gaps with temporary employees. This lack of cohesion on the part of the staff and leadership causes residents with dementia to experience more anxiety and confusion than their condition itself produces.

Even residents' families feel called upon to help in some situations. We do not want them to have to do that. Their role is to be there for their family member, not to be constantly letting the director know about the problems with the home, or chasing down a staff member to change a resident's incontinence pad.

One of the biggest problems at many nursing homes is a lack of strong leaders who dare to challenge the system. Along the same lines, a care home cannot be led according to a leadership theory, a management template, or a master's degree thesis. When I observe Dagmarsminde, and everything going on there—the residents, their families, and my colleagues—it is like watching the open sea. My job is to keep the waves rising, breaking, and crashing with the least amount of ripple. The only way I can do it is if I am driven by a call.

Objection:
"We have to follow state regulations."

Large nursing home systems, whether public or privately run, are full of lists, instructions, jargon, and templates for doing things: "multidisciplinary approach"; "aerobic exercise for aging brains"; "visitation guidelines for relatives"; "Dementia Package–3"; "home health care"; "activating, rehabilitating, and compensating strategies"; "the five levels of ability." Procedures and rules for moving residents into the home or for making food, such as "Don't put food where the residents can reach," have the goal of making the care home a "safe work environment." The main focus of these efforts is the staff, not the residents. And if the focus switches to the residents, then they are grouped by their functional ability levels and categorized accordingly, enabling the staff to divide up the help and attention each will receive. It is obviously a little difficult to think creatively and freely in this kind of environment.

Following the Rules, but with the Focus on Residents

Dagmarsminde is a different world. We have to meet county regulations, but at the same time, in order to enable our work, we have to distance ourselves from restrictive frameworks, break free of them when we can. First, we look at the rules. What are they? What if they have been interpreted to suit a certain way of working? Maybe they could be interpreted differently, in a way that reveals new possibilities.

Under normal circumstances, employees can become obsessed with interpreting everything as protocol—for what they cannot do. This is a negative perspective, which hinders them from developing. Sometimes we have to look twice to see whether a rule is a *mandate* or a *recommendation*. If it is a recommendation, we begin by interpreting it in a way that fits with what we want to accomplish. Obviously, this means having staff and leadership who are brave enough to interpret the rules and make them suit the values of their home.

Rigid protocols exist throughout the nursing home industry, and often these do not appear to be related to the core value of protecting the well-being of the residents. I recently read a regulation that specified how staff were not allowed to move their residents "vertically"—only "horizontally." The regulation called for a "zero-tolerance policy," which means that the staff were prohibited from offering a resident their hand to help the person get up from a chair. Staff were not even allowed to touch the residents who could not get up by themselves.

In other words, the staff always had to use a lift. When a resident fell down, he stayed on the floor until they could find a lift to pick him up. I saw this with my own eyes when I visited a public nursing home as a consultant. In that case, it so happened the battery had run out on the lift, so the staff brought out a sheet they could use to drag the elderly gentleman, who had severe dementia, across the floor all the way to his room. Once there, they hooked him up to the apparatus, which lifted him into bed, where they examined him for bruises or injuries. It was degrading for the poor man.

These rules, imposed for work health and safety considerations, are created in the interest of the staff and, ostensibly, the residents, but they often are most beneficial for the organization. If the focus had been on the resident, three employees might have carefully lifted the man up; at least he would have felt as if he were receiving the same help if he had fallen on the sidewalk. Instead, he was treated as if he had the plague and dragged across the floor in plain view, to the horror of the other residents. This left the man feeling both embarrassed and alienated. That is hardly conducive to building that all-important bond that is essential for the residents to feel safe at their most vulnerable.

The only way to stamp out this kind of rigid protocol is if both directors and employees collectively oppose them. If a rule does not ensure the residents the care they need, then we should resist abiding by them and work to change them. As health professionals, we need to be prepared to argue why a particular instruction might do more harm than good.

In Denmark at least, these kinds of guidelines are usually formulated by people at the county offices or others in leadership positions who are far removed from day-to-day care. Whenever possible, I believe the staff who work closely with residents must take responsibility for calling out regulations that hinder them from caring in their care work. If the regulation cannot be changed, make the effort to work creatively within that system to find solutions that benefit the residents in your care.

Care home residents with dementia need to be
surrounded by people who can perceive how they are
doing and what needs they have here and now.

Summary

We should not run our care homes according to a standardized set of rules. We are working with people who have very specific, individual needs. When we have to move these people, and help them feel better, we should not think only in terms of protocol. Care home residents with dementia need to be surrounded by people who can perceive how they are doing and what needs they have here and now. They need to be cared for by employees who are willing to engage on a personal level, and who draw on their own experiences and ideas for the best solution, as if they were in that situation themselves. Trust and openness are essential between the resident and each individual staff member, and that bond should not be derailed by protocol.

Therefore, I encourage you to look for opportunities to break free. If you want to work according to your own discretion and feeling for your craft and respond to the deep-rooted call to care for those who need it, then dig in your heels where you can. Define your own values and let them guide you toward connection and resourcefulness at your care home. If you are in a system with strict rules and protocols, try to work creatively within that system with your focus always on the resident's best interest. This focus can work like a spell—a sprinkling of stardust over the residents—which only happens when we have trust in both ourselves and each other.

———— •◆• ————

Questions for Reflection

1. Consider the author's discussion of "the selfless workplace" and "call to service." To what extent do you share these values,

and to what extent does your own workplace encourage and express them?

2. Imagine you are a resident of the care home in which you are presently working, or where you have worked previously. What are some ways in which the staff seem more or less focused on their own needs compared to yours? List some contrasts in the different experiences of care.

3. Is there a process or procedure at your workplace that you believe could be carried out in a more person-centered way? Consider why it is done the way it is; if you feel it should change, what are the obstacles?

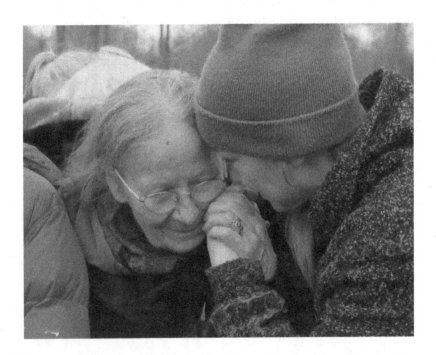

5

· ◆ ·

Tapering Off Medication

Purification and Stability

ONE OF OUR DRIVING PRINCIPLES here at Dagmarsminde is to replace medicine with care. In other words care, not medicine, is our treatment. I feel strongly about this issue because medicine can cause so many problems for nursing home residents who suffer from dementia. I believe it is wrong to dull the senses of people with dementia by using heavy doses of medicine, and I have made this point on many different platforms: in my first book, in newspapers, on television, in panels, and on radio programs. Medicating like this is simply oppressive.

Tapering medication, by contrast, can be a purifying process that stabilizes the resident's mental and physical strength. This process enables us to reach the real, original human being, which is also the starting ground for our care work. That is how we prepare the resident for the nourishment we wish to offer him or her, helping the person put down roots and grow new branches.

Working with Existing Prescriptions

The majority of new residents at Danish nursing homes move in with a suitcase full of pills. Many of them have been given a dangerous cocktail of different medications over the years, without knowledge of the consequences of these pharmaceutical concoctions. What is clear is that the effects and side effects of these medications can partially obscure the resident's actual condition. In addition, an older person's kidneys may have a difficult time expelling the medicine, which can gradually accumulate in the body.

This seemingly indiscriminate approach to medication in the field of dementia, an almost-automatic prescribing of drugs, testifies to a culture shaped by a mechanized and impatient world, one that is focused on immediate solutions. It is imperative we stop the hasty use of medicine in our attempts to improve the residents' quality of life.

Below is a suggested sequence for tapering off the kinds of medicines new residents usually have on their prescription lists. The process is actually easier than one might think, as long as the staff at the nursing home are prepared to surround the resident with attentive, loving care and natural sensory experiences.

Tapering Sequence

The moment we first sit down with a resident's prescription list, we look at the scope of drugs involved and start thinking about how to taper them. As the person gets his or her bearings in new surroundings, which could take days or weeks, the new resident continues taking the prescribed drugs. As soon as possible, we review the prescription list with the general practitioner for our home.

Here, I would like to highlight the importance of having a physician we can consult with on a regular basis. Our doctor is familiar with, and sympathetic to, the fundamental values of the care home while also understanding the issues involved with drug interactions and overmedication.

Sleeping pills

We start with the sleeping pills, followed by sedatives and antipsychotics. What is the alternative for sleeping pills, sedatives, and antipsychotics? Nothing, other than the resident's new routine. First and foremost, we address the sleep cycle by not letting residents stay in bed all day. They need to sleep at night. We find that people with dementia need a lot of sleep, including a good night's sleep of at least 11 to 13 hours. Beyond that, naps are necessary throughout the day. In the remaining time periods, the residents need to stay active in order to feel tired in the evening. I describe this in more detail in Chapter 9, where circadian rhythms are discussed.

Addressing sleep issues

Sleep is a way for the body to restore itself. It enables all of us to reduce stress and prepare for new experiences. We believe people are better off not using sleeping pills, even if they have trouble sleeping. When people take sleeping pills, the resulting sleep is less deep than its natural counterpart, and they are more likely to wake up in the night. This is where the problem arises; it is difficult to go back to sleep after that. People with dementia really need a natural, deep sleep, with dreams that are not affected by medicine.

The residents at Dagmarsminde do not usually have problems sleeping. Most of them sleep really well. There are, of course, instances when someone might wake up at night, but we do not administer sleeping pills for that. We simply consider why the person is waking up and address that issue. The first step to implementing this strategy is to make sure the resident's chart does not include "PRN" (as needed) instructions for medications in their charts. Working this way, in consultation with our physician, we eliminate the possibility of a resident being given a sleeping pill before other strategies are attempted. There is always a reason why people wake up in the middle of the night, and our first step is to try to discover that reason.

Life at Our Home

One of our residents had itchy skin, which would waken him feeling frustrated and unable to fall back asleep. We put our heads together and tried different lotions and methods. We did not give up. We figured out the exact number of times to apply lotion, swabbed him with a cloth, and aired out the room in order to diminish his symptoms. The point is, our practice is to react immediately to any changes in residents who usually sleep throughout the night. Some situations take more work than others. But we figure it out.

It is important to note that we have two staff members on our night shift, whereas many care homes deprioritize the necessity for staff at night. This is a mistake that has a serious impact on the residents' well-being. Getting a good night's sleep is just as crucial for them as it is for the rest of us. This is why we make an extra effort to ensure a calm and peaceful environment when a resident wakes up in the middle of the night.

Every night, one or more of our residents will undoubtedly wake up and feel confused. In all the years since Dagmarsminde opened, however, we do not respond by giving a sleeping pill. We head to the resident's room as soon as we notice they are out of bed, either because their room sensor lets us know or—for those who do not have a sensor in their room—when they come out to us in the living room. We speak quietly to the person who is awake and make it clear that it is nighttime and everyone is asleep. We ascertain whether he or she needs to go to the bathroom, the room is too warm or too cold, the sheet or down comforter has gathered uncomfortably, or there are any other disturbing conditions. Then we sit and calmly talk to the resident. Within 10 minutes, the person is usually fast asleep again.

Of course some will have a harder time going back to sleep. In those cases, what often works is making them a little snack— for example, a slice of bread and cheese along with a cup of chamomile tea or other calming herbal tea with milk. This can help the resident feel comforted, cared for, and more "whole" again. In these situations, we take on a kind of mothering role. Another good trick is the company of our cat on the resident's bed.

Sedatives and antipsychotics

After we have tapered the resident's sleeping medications, we turn our attention to any sedatives or antipsychotics he or she has been taking, which were undoubtedly prescribed to alleviate anxiety and restlessness. Health authorities the world over increasingly recommend that these medications not be given to people with dementia, in part because of the many side effects, and in part because the drugs have not proven effective in people with dementia. The agitated states that often lead to the prescription of these drugs are usually triggered by the individual's reaction to an environment that does not meet their needs rather than an internal physical disturbance. For instance, an uneasy state might be due to a problem with the person's hearing aid.

In another example, a person with dementia might perceive a room and objects within it differently from those of us without dementia. The resident might think he or she sees something or will point at something that does not exist for the rest of us. Hallucinations are among the symptoms of dementia, and—contrary to practices in many nursing homes—usually need not be treated with drugs. The resident may not actually be experiencing any discomfort from his or her alternative perception of the room or object. In most cases, an acknowledgment of the person and his or her own perceptions, combined with the right activities, is "treatment" enough.

Anti-anxiety and antipsychotic drugs have to be slowly tapered. A hurried tapering only heightens the risk of the individual becoming more anxious. For all medications, the doctor evaluates the rate of tapering together with the staff who work with the resident on a daily basis. The staff and doctor assess the resident's condition throughout the tapering process and even after it has concluded.

Antidepressants

We begin tapering antidepressants, which are oddly prescribed to almost everyone with a dementia diagnosis, once
a new resident appears settled. The resident needs to feel at
ease here before any medication reductions are started. Many
with dementia are given antidepressants because the diagnosis
itself can trigger a sense of hopelessness, a fear of humiliation
and loss of control, and a feeling of not fitting in anymore. It is
understandable that the doctor would try to ease this so-called
depression to prevent the patient from giving up. Yet the sadness rooted in the decline of one's identity cannot be altered by
medication, unless the drug is so strong the person ends up in
a vegetative state. Dementia represents a complete transformation of one's life, an existential crisis, in which a person needs
professional help to mentally process the situation and find his
or her bearings. For me, it is clear that changes in one's personality should be handled on a human level and not chemically.
The emotional downturn is so complex that only the interaction
between another complex human mind and the person's mind
can relieve the suffering.

People with dementia who are on antidepressants—
sometimes two different kinds—can seem utterly deflated
and indifferent to the world around them. Some will have a
higher threshold than others, but I believe these people are
better off being able to experience the profoundness of their
feelings so that, together with their care partners, they can
work through their crisis and pass through to another, newer
side of life.

We believe it is healthy for the resident to huddle and
cry for a time, and then reach out for consolation. Often, that
is the moment we open up to each other and gain a deeper
understanding of the resident. Allowing for this understanding will benefit the resident in other circumstances, such as
when we need to interpret a sign from him or her or alleviate
a discomfort. Every time a resident reacts and reveals difficult
emotions, we gain valuable knowledge. The same goes for the

opposite situation, when a resident—without the dulling effect of antidepressants—suddenly bursts into laughter, gets up, dances around, and squeezes the cheeks of a staff member and embraces them. The apathy is gone. The point is: The only way we can help the resident live with his or her condition is if the road to understanding it is not blocked by medicine. Once that is gone, we have a chance to read the person's expression and to experience the outbursts of anger or the "I don't want tos" as well as the moments of enthusiasm.

Antidepressants have numerous side effects beyond just the undesirable dulling effect. These include fatigue, nausea, stomach cramps, shaking, and insomnia—problems that we do not want to add to the already complicated life people with dementia face on an everyday basis. We have to remember that a resident with severe dementia may be unable to communicate an experience of nausea. Instead, the person may just stay in bed and stop eating, which leaves him or her without the energy to do even the smallest things. This daily exhaustion can also mean the resident does not make it to the bathroom. It is not a good situation for anyone, but the person may not understand that his or her suffering is caused by the side effects of medicine. At the same time, he or she may be unable to communicate a specific discomfort like needing to go to the bathroom.

To understand what it is like for a resident on one of these anti-anxiety medications, imagine a person tucked under a duvet, wrapped too tightly to be able to respond to any kind of stimulation. If he or she has been heavily medicated, the "duvet" will be even heavier. When we taper the medication, we are lifting off the blanket, exposing the person to a wave of sensory experience like a sudden waft of cold air. Having to absorb so many new impressions can trigger restlessness and physical exhaustion. Therefore, we have to be prepared to see the resident struggle as the body fights to stabilize. We need to be attentive and allow enough time for natural balance to be restored. The reaction will not be strong as long we stay close by and include the person in community life, while also allowing for relaxation by not requiring constant participation. There is not a set procedure, as every case is unique, but as long as we understand the cold-air metaphor, as staff members working in concert with a medical professional and other staff, we can minimize the "drafts" through human interaction and other natural methods.

Pain relievers

Our new residents often have one thing in common: They are used to taking painkillers. Paracetamol (also known as acetaminophen or Tylenol) can appear on their medicine chart three or four times a day. When a resident takes 3 grams of paracetamol on a daily basis over 3 years, it means 3,285 grams of the medication pass through their body for no reason.

Painkillers are administered to people with dementia because they often express discomfort as an expression of feeling powerless. If their previous surroundings failed to address the problem, painkillers were only an arm's length away. Doctors in those settings may not have explored the actual origin of the pain because of time constraints.

When our new residents arrive with pain relievers on their list and we do not know the concrete reason for it—such as a fracture, arthritis, or the like—we try to figure out the reason through trial and error. Aided by our physician, we stop the pain relievers and see what ensues. Usually, nothing alarming happens. As we accommodate residents and their emotional needs, and they begin to feel a purpose within the new context, nothing triggers the pain. We see it time and again.

We have stopped the use of morphine, arthritis medicine, and paracetamol in this way. Suddenly, residents who have regained their speech are not battling stomach cramps anymore, and on the whole are drawn out of an unnecessary victimhood. Also, when the residents are not given pain relievers throughout the day, it is easier for us to assess when they actually have a headache or a backache, which may require a pain reliever. We become more acutely attuned to their symptoms. Residents should have acetaminophen when they need it, of course, as for a headache or foot pain that can trigger a strong reaction. Generally, though, we believe that drugs for pain relief should not be on the resident's list of regular medications.

Anti-hypertensive medications

Many of our new residents are on drugs for high blood pressure, also known as anti-hypertensive medication. This type of medication often leads to nausea, stomach cramps, blurred vision, coughing, an altered sense of taste, shortness of breath, and depression, just to mention a few of the side effects. The person with dementia will have difficulty communicating the presence of any of these side effects. Instead, we often see the resident reacting by eating too little or becoming anxious, angry, or withdrawn. Once again, the side effects can trigger the dementia symptoms that staff find challenging. As of this writing, with help from our physician as well as close monitoring, we have successfully tapered all high blood pressure medication previously prescribed to our residents.

Diuretics

Diuretics are commonly prescribed for older adults, mostly for lowering blood pressure or for preventing fluid retention. The most common side effects of these drugs are dizziness, due to lowered blood pressure, and constipation, resulting from all the fluids having been washed out of their intestines. To counter the latter side effect, laxatives are often prescribed, leading to the potential for more side effects.

More often than not, we can remove the diuretic medication, or at least reduce it, without causing any life-threatening complications. The resident's urination usually becomes more controlled and regular. It also becomes easier to maintain the body's fluid balance so the resident's bowel movements return to normal. When we take away the diuretic, the basic bodily functions usually return to normal.

Other medications

In a similar fashion—always in consultation with our physician—
we begin removing other medications that are considered almost
sacred, such as heart-rhythm stabilizers, also known as blood-
thinning or anti-cramping drugs. Parkinson's medications can
also be scaled back or stopped completely.

The many possibilities for tapering medication are often
overlooked. Yet one thing is clear to me: The human body was
not designed to need medication. Scientific development has
enabled us to cure diseases and alleviate discomfort, which is
wonderful. But offering more nuanced care and nursing for the
vulnerable, who can neither address their own symptoms nor
care for their own well-being, and who are in the final phase of
their lives, means carefully considering everything that might
affect their quality of life.

I could spend more time on the side effects of different
medications, but my suggestion is that every time you evaluate a resident's medication, research the most common side
effects. Although most medicine has undesirable effects on just
1%–10% of users, some have side effects that affect more than
10% of those who take them. This includes Alzheimer medication as well, which is the last category I will cover.

Medication for dementia

A person who is diagnosed with dementia is often immediately
prescribed Alzheimer's medication, such as donepezil (also
known as Aricept). The medication is often presented as the
only solution, and therefore a kind of salvation. No one refuses
the possibility of recovery, of course, but it is misleading to suggest the medicine can stop the progression of the disease. It
works for a while, but unfortunately, its actual effect or how
long it lasts is still uncertain.

The medication enables some people to maintain their
abilities or even slightly improve, whereas others only experience the side effects. Yet the common denominator for all
Alzheimer's drugs developed so far is that their effect does not

seem to be permanent. Many only see a change for a couple of months. Apparently, donepezil has been proven most effective if taken at the onset of dementia. It is worth asking, then, why medication for Alzheimer's disease would even be used at a care home, where the residents are usually in the more advanced phases of the illness.

Donepezil is widely used to treat Alzheimer's disease, Lewy body dementia, and Parkinson's disease. In consultation with our physician, we have decided never to administer it in our care home, where the target group of those with mild to moderate dementia is relatively small. Below, I point out the most common side effects of this drug. It is helpful to connect these side effects with what we already know about the stress, anxiety, and other difficulties experienced by a person with severe dementia.

Following are the most common side effects, which occur in more than 10% of patients who take donepezil:

- Diarrhea
- Nausea
- Headaches

Other common side effects, occurring in up to 10% of those who take the medicine, include:

- Reduced appetite
- Pains
- Fatigue
- Abnormal dreams
- Aggression
- Agitation
- Hallucinations
- Dizziness
- Insomnia
- Irritable skin
- Incontinence

Are we willing to expose the resident to these kinds of discomforts? Yes, if we are 100% sure that the person's life will improve with donepezil. We are obligated to find out, on the resident's behalf, and we can do this by gradually reducing the drug in consultation with the doctor. Anything else would be irresponsible.

Another medication our new residents have often been taking before they arrive at Dagmarsminde is memantine, which is prescribed for moderate to severe Alzheimer's disease. Again, it is helpful to consider each of the following side effects—to stop and reflect on each one—in relation to the challenges the resident already faces on a daily basis as a result of his or her dementia.

Following are examples of common side effects of memantine that occur in up to 10% of patients:

- Constipation
- Problems breathing/shortness of breath
- Fatigue
- Balance issues
- Headaches
- Dizziness
- Hypersensitivity

It can be very difficult to assess the effect of Alzheimer's drugs, and when we consider this difficulty along with the amount of time a resident has left to live, I urge more caution regarding the widespread use of these drugs. I realize how frightening it must be to eliminate that last glimmer of hope that the medicine represents for many relatives. Because of this fear, it is easy to turn a blind eye to the side effects. I also realize that some people with dementia will not experience any side effects. But before completely abandoning the idea of removing the medicine, we should at least double-check that the medicine actually has a positive effect and that the effect is not eclipsed by its side effects. If nothing else, cultivating these kinds of questions may lead to a more judicious and well-founded use of strong medications.

We usually wait to taper the Alzheimer's drugs until we have weaned the resident off other medicines entirely. As the resident settles into the new care environment and no longer shows any side effects from the other drugs, we gain a clearer picture of the person's actual dementia symptoms. We often notice the resident having fewer negative and sudden reactions. The previous erratic behavior was a result of the drug-induced side effects and the way the person was perceived and treated over a long period. Combined with a long list of chemically induced physical discomforts, he or she may have felt misunderstood, different, isolated, or alienated.

Once we are happy with our professional assessment of the situation, it is time to gradually taper the Alzheimer's medication. It is my experience that the residents get better. They perk up and become more open. For some, we even see an improvement in their abilities. We have also seen residents for whom there were *no* signs of improvement after we tapered the Alzheimer's medication. Their condition did not change, but even in these cases, it did not make sense to continue the drugs.

I would like to add one last important factor regarding the tapering of Alzheimer's medicine. Taking away this supposed "last solution" affects our perspective. We begin seeking new solutions and ways to improve the residents' abilities and to make life easier for them. The removal of the medication forces us to draw on our creativity and our human strengths to benefit the lives of our residents. This is where our work becomes challenging and inspiring as we go to great lengths for them.

Broadly speaking, I advocate checking whether the benefit of a medicine is indisputable, or if the side effects pose a greater risk and are essentially detrimental to the resident's quality of life. Even something as simple as receiving two or three pills every morning can have a negative effect on a resident's quality of life. The person asks, "What are those for? Why do I need to take them?" Additionally, it can be difficult to administer the medication—getting it into the resident's mouth and ensuring a pill is properly swallowed—because the person with dementia may have a hard time contracting the esophagus. The decision to prescribe medication should take into consideration that the resident of a care home may only have months or a very few years left to live. It is an ethical question to use or remove medication. Nursing care without an emphasis on medication allows us to include more of this ethical dimension in our treatment.

Support for Healthy Living

When tapering medications, it is important to provide as much support as possible for the resident's good overall health. We provide food with fresh ingredients full of important vitamins and minerals, help the residents get some fresh air, and offer plenty of opportunities to stimulate both the body and mind on a daily basis. These efforts help the residents to improve from within. They start feeling more comfortable in their own skin, in touch with their senses, and for the first time in a while, self-aware. Each person is somebody who matters and is still a part of this world. Perhaps a resident will become what is often described as "unfiltered"—will start complaining or making more demands. This is not necessarily "just the disease speaking"; it is the person *behind* the disease, who has awakened and has wants and needs. To go back to the roots/tree metaphor, which I used at the start of this chapter, once we have helped the person put down roots and grow new branches, we should be glad when he or she can ask us for water.

So-called unfiltered communication can actually be a healthy sign that the resident understands we are here for his or her sake. It is an opening, a sign of trust. When new residents come to the care home, it can take at least a couple of months for them to feel at ease, to feel good, and to actively participate—in their own way and with their own individual vulnerabilities, which of course vary from person to person.

The wonderful thing about a care home is that we have the possibility of creating the necessary conditions for good health after tapering medications. Tapering in any shape or form requires stability, caring, and understanding.

The Norm:
"Let's give these drugs a shot."

The treatment culture at most Danish nursing homes, as well as in many other places in the world, is to try medicine first. Putting it plainly, the pill is seen as the first solution to all problems. Have you seen this at your care home? As soon as you mention that a resident tends to burst out crying, he or she is swiftly prescribed an antidepressant to "curb it." The doctor may dial the medicine dosage up or down or replace one pill with another. This mechanized approach might make sense for a medical team treating an acute condition in a hospital, but it does not belong at a care home with vulnerable people who have dementia. The resident's situation does not allow for a constant adjustment of chemicals for an immediate effect.

Undoubtedly, the doctor and staff only have the best intentions with every new drug, but when dealing with people with dementia, good intentions are useless without thoroughly evaluating our actions. There are so many ethical questions to consider when working with these people. The balance of power is skewed on different levels because they have dementia and we do not. It is up to us as professionals or relatives to let our doubt be to the benefit of the ones in our care who have dementia.

Some ethical questions to ask in order to decide whether or not to try a new drug on a resident are the following:

- Does the resident understand what the medicine is for?
- Does the person understand the possible side effects?
- Is the person able to communicate his or her experience of side effects?
- Can the person communicate the effectiveness of the medication?

- How does the new pill work or interact with other medications the person may be taking?
- Do the resident's kidneys expel the medicine or will it accumulate?
- Can the resident administer the medicine without help from others? If not, will you have to hide it in his or her food?
- Does the person's throat hurt when swallowing pills?
- Do the pills affect the person's appetite, so that he or she does not eat enough?

It is important to see how these questions—and countless more— touch upon how bearable or unbearable potential side effects may be. So, no, we should not just "give these drugs a shot." It is a serious decision, which on a basic moral level requires a more thorough examination than is usually allowed for.

Bearing in mind all the factors involved in considering a new drug for someone with dementia, it is striking how quick doctors are to prescribe them. I believe all health professionals shirk from responsibility when they do not take a stance on either the new or the current drugs administered. It is not because they are indifferent or do not care about the people in their care; they are simply victims of the same "medicated daze" that has affected all of us as a society—potentially at the expense of older adults and their quality of life.

Objection:
"There's a reason they developed the medicine!"

If a person is in a constant state of suffering from the side effects of a single medication or combination of drugs—nausea, dizziness, headaches, and so on—then obviously, even with the best intentions, we are going to have a hard time reaching them. In other words, the medicine hampers our work. We can try to love and care for them as much as we like, but it will not make a difference.

Voices from the ailing culture of care unanimously declare, "There is a reason they developed the medicine. The people get sick." Yes, sometimes they get sick. For example, they get urinary tract infections, which require antibiotics. But in regard to the challenges the residents face, such as anxiety, sadness, and insomnia, we have other methods for addressing these issues. It is what the staff, the ones caring for the residents, were originally trained for. Human relations, activities, exercises, caring, and nursing can be effective replacements for medicine in people with dementia.

I have already mentioned how the majority of the medicines the residents receive often end up not making any difference. We can only find that out when we dare to remove them, not before. We may give residents pain relievers every day over a long period and report: "I can see the pills are working because he doesn't feel any pain." We can make the same assessment on the following days, weeks, and months. In a similar vein, we might say, "The Parkinson's drugs must be working because her body is just as stiff today as it was yesterday, when she got the same dose."

The default position should not be to use medication. First and foremost, we should be advocating for how the person is faring, and how they might fare, without it. Relatives have told me that if they wanted to try pausing the Alzheimer's medication being given to their loved one, they often have had to come prepared with counter-arguments before talking to the doctor. It is as though the culture has decided the elderly patient is more manageable when medicated.

Summary

Tapering medication is often presented as being risky and unsafe, which is why we need to speak out, present our strong counter-arguments, and provide careful documentation and evaluation when we implement a change. This takes courage. Courageous administrators and employees have to stand their ground and signal that this is the plan now. We must dare to take a different path that offers a fresh outlook and forces us to think harder, to talk to each other, to listen to each other's observations, and to notice subtle divergences in the resident's condition and work on them. This is how we start, by critically evaluating the list of medications, discussing them with the doctor at least once a month, and gradually clearing them out, one by one. All the while, we must boost the remaining health of the resident with good food, appropriate exercise, great company, and excellent care.

———— •◆• ————

Questions for Reflection

1. What do you think about the policies and practices described in this chapter?

2. How do the policies in your workplace regarding use of medications compare with the policies described in this chapter?

3. Do you think any changes in medication policies in your care home should be considered? Why or why not?

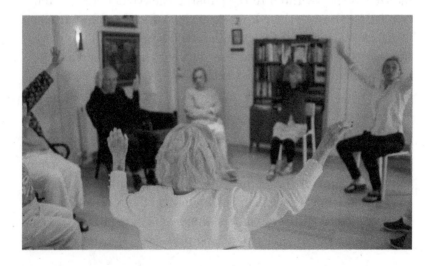

6

·◆·

Exercise:

Active Residents Seize the Day

ANYONE CAN EXERCISE. ANYONE CAN have a goal and feel good about getting better at something. Staff at care homes can help residents improve their physical strength, their attitude toward it, and their belief in their own abilities. In this chapter, I present some different ways of exercising with residents at a care home, starting with basic physical exercises and training.

Readers may wonder why I use the word "training," rather than the oft-used care term "rehabilitation," which might seem nicer and more sympathetic in regard to the resident's cognitive and physical abilities. Here is the distinction:

- *Training* implies moving forward, developing new skills, and meeting new goals—practicing at activities that one has the ability to do.

- *Rehabilitation* implies fixing something from the past or returning to some normal state of the past, compensating for a disability.

Training, in this sense, is more optimistic. We are not here just to maintain the resident's condition and prevent further decline. We set optimistic goals, and we try to keep the morale of the staff as well as the residents high in order to reach as many of them as we can. Our target for any resident, no matter how frail he or she may be, is to reach our goals together. We may or may not succeed. But we try, and—successful or not—we find a new goal. This is not about obtaining specific results, but about finding the courage and spirit to do the training. We keep the resident's physical condition and abilities in mind at all times. When the person finally becomes old and tired, and so weak that there is no point in training any longer, then we can feel confident that we tried our best. Before that point, there is a way, and there is change. This is the movement we are looking for when we think of training.

It is important to read the following examples for training as *suggestions* for what can be done. I am presenting what has worked at Dagmarsminde. Training at other care homes might be different. How training is organized at any home depends on the cultural framework of the home and the condition of the residents. Activities need to suit the individual, but our basic principle is that no goal is too high. I invite you to consider the ideas in this chapter optimistically, with even some of your weakest residents in mind.

Expectation as Inspiration

After years of inactivity, many new residents need to recover their physical strength. Some—perhaps out of habit—can be a little lazy about it. That probably sounds harsh, but they have, perhaps unwittingly, been allowed to be stationary for too long. At Dagmarsminde, we ask the residents to "grab life by the horns," without spending too much time complaining about it being too hard. If the staff's gung-ho attitude says, "Let's get going!" the residents will follow. Often, we see a difference in their willingness to move after only a couple of days. It is good for the new resident to feel we have high expectations. Having expectations of others is one way of saying we value them. Our approach is not just an upbeat pep talk, it is more like a tender well-wishing; after all, we are on this journey with them.

Life at Our Home

Residents who move to Dagmarsminde from other care homes bring with them a set of medical or nursing notes—a journal—that provides background on their condition. The journal of one of our residents indicated that she was unable to walk more than a couple of steps. But from the moment she arrived at Dagmarsminde, we welcomed her with our optimism. She walked right in the main door and continued into the shared living space, where she stalwartly paced the room, saying: "What a nice place." The staff's energy and trusting smiles seemed to contradict her negative self-image as someone with "decreased mobility." She felt like moving.

As I have mentioned previously, many of the drugs prescribed to the residents are the very reason they are physically hampered when they first arrive. Many of them experience shortness of breath moving around, or feel nauseous and dizzy—and so, understandably, prefer not to move. By building up their confidence and encouraging them to believe in themselves from day one, we motivate them. When we begin tapering the medicine, we experience an additional push in the right direction. They will go the distance.

Motivate for Movement

In general, our first rule is to motivate the new resident from day one to be more active. In reality, it is more about faith than motivation. We show the residents we believe in them from the moment they set foot in our care home. How that looks will vary from home to home. There is no reason to roll out the red carpet with excitement, but it might help for staff and leadership to consider the kind of signal they want the home to send to the new resident.

At the kind of care home we strive to create, daily exercise is among our core values, and that should be evident to the residents and relatives from the start. At Dagmarsminde, all of the residents participate in our activity program on a daily basis. This begins with 1 hour of group exercises. We also walk outdoors in the fresh air, feed and tend the animals, or move around in our warm-water pool.

The residents are on the move from the start, often moving more than they did at home, and they are exhausted by the end of the day. Their bodies might ache, in the same way our own muscles and joints would ache if we spontaneously ran 5 miles. That does not mean we automatically reach for the painkillers for the residents. The solution to aching muscles could be massage. Or sometimes it is enough to explain that their soreness is from exercising, which is healthy and good; most of them understand this.

> *We show the residents we believe in them from the moment they set foot in our care home.*

Residents never overtly express the desire to be inactive. At the start, many of them fall back into the role of being old and not needing to move. But as soon as we get them going, they accept that movement is a part of their new daily routine. Then the same thing happens that happens to anyone else who exercises: They get happier and stronger. Then—quiet as mice—we raise the bar, subtly increasing their daily exercise.

Walking

At Dagmarsminde, residents have to walk to everything, even if only a short distance. They walk from the chair to the sofa, from the living room to the bathroom, or from their own room to the shared living space. We aim for as many steps as possible.

Group Exercise

Beyond walking, we lead the residents in group exercises that focus on individual muscle groups. Sometimes we use resistance bands, hand weights, or the body's own weight. We do not have a lot of gym and fitness equipment or a specialized room. We usually exercise in the shared living spaces. Our program is simple and straightforward. Once in a while, a physical therapist visits and shows us some new techniques or helps train with individual residents.

However, we do not rely on having a physical therapist. Our regular staff can lead the exercises or invent new creative ways to move. We are not trying to train our residents in technique for the next marathon or athletic competition. We may invite them to move in ways that are based on our own experience and inspiration. We invite the residents to swing their arms back and forth, stretch their necks, stomp on the floor, or throw a ball. We have all had gym at school, and plenty of fitness information is available to us today if we need ideas.

The shape of our shared morning exercises depends on who is leading them. The individual staff member invents the movements. We usually arrange a circle of chairs in the middle of our shared living space, and the activity is performed to a playlist of cheerful, familiar tunes in different tempos. One of our favorite exercises is called "Get Up–Sit Down." The residents have to get up and sit down in their chairs; some do the exercise squatting down while holding onto the back of the chair. Throughout the exercises, we raise the bar: "Yesterday you did three, try doing four," and so on. This is one of our most important exercises because it strengthens the residents' core muscle groups and improves their balance when they stand up, thus enabling them to get up on their own. By the end, we are all breaking a sweat, which brings a smile to our faces.

Weight training also takes place in our shared living space, with all of us sitting in a circle. We do a combination of muscle training and coordination exercises. We also lead the residents in cardiovascular exercise, which can be either dancing or an exercise where they hold the back of a chair and stretch their legs in different directions. For coordination training, we might practice crossing our arms and legs in various patterns; this is also a mental challenge. In addition, we usually have the residents recite a rhyme throughout the activity.

We also lead residents in sensory training, inviting them to pat their arms, legs, and face. This helps them to gain an awareness of their own body and at the same time increases their circulation. In between the exercises, the instructor stops the music and leads a memory exercise, asking each resident to sit in the circle, say their name, and tell the group what kind of work they did in the past. This is an exercise in validating each person, which creates a nice atmosphere of friendship, solidarity, and team spirit. Each resident in the circle becomes more than just another care home resident to the others.

For the weakest residents who cannot walk and never will because of the advanced phase of their illness, we help them do exercises in bed. We start every morning by moving their legs, pelvis, and back, activating their entire body. Even though they exercise in bed, these residents have a seat at our shared exercise hour, so they can absorb the energy from the other residents and feel included.

Some residents benefit from either walking or running on our treadmill. The treadmill is especially useful for the active residents, who might otherwise restlessly pace the floors with their abundance of energy. They entirely forget their lost abilities once they jump on the treadmill. Staff members can adjust the incline for climbing—the function we use most often—to stimulate more muscle groups. Usually, residents who have been exercising on the treadmill are proud of themselves and, to our amusement, will insist on having broken their previous record.

We also train residents in our warm-water pool; the warm water increases their circulation. Some of the residents enjoy being in the water more than others. For those who get a taste for relaxing in the warm water, it works wonders for their condition. It is not unusual for someone to ask first thing in the morning if there is time for a swim in the "big bathtub."

The person on the night shift may even slip into the water with the resident before the shift is done.

For the residents who enjoy it, spending time in the water helps release endorphins. The resident might float or stand in the water, supported by a staff member who leads him or her through various exercises depending on the resident's capabilities. Afterwards, there is a relaxation session. Sometimes, a resident will fall asleep with his or her head on the staff member's shoulder. The warm water, together with the skin-to-skin contact, offers stimulation on many levels.

Moving as a Way of Life

Beyond having daily shared cardiovascular exercises, it is important to also have high standards when it comes to the physical needs of each individual resident. So, in between the shared sessions, we ensure each resident is moving according to his or her own needs. This might include climbing stairs, yoga, or exercising to strengthen the stomach muscles or an ankle that needs stabilizing. All of this is possible, even for those residents who had previously sat stooped over all day long. The combination of their increased confidence, daily training, and the simple act of walking from place to place not only increases their strength, it naturally wears them out and they sleep better at night. They need it. We make sure to incorporate training in every activity. Even putting on shoes can be training. Residents have to bend over to tie their laces, first one and then the other. After they have been to the toilet, they have to pull up their pants, walk over to the sink, and wash their hands. We also encourage residents to lend a hand with the daily tasks of our care home, which uses their bodies in all sorts of small ways throughout the day.

Training is one of our core values at Dagmarsminde. It is an integral part of every day. The residents need to anticipate and count on doing some sort of physical exercise—today. And I can attest to the fact that they do. Even at breakfast, a couple of them will always ask, "Is it time for aerobics?"

Screening

Training the residents for their different abilities means regularly screening the residents as well. We use the Alzheimer's Disease Cooperative Study–Activities of Daily Living Scale[1,2] (ADCS-ADL Scale) to evaluate their abilities. We carry out the assessment every other month so we can track each resident's development, making sure both the day and evening teams run the test to get the most valid results. Afterward, we calculate the average results and list the resident's score on a graph. We measure their basic abilities, which for people with dementia are usually impaired. The screening includes everything from bathing to taking out the trash, from making coffee to understanding how to use a phone, being alone, and so on.

We notice notice that many of the residents, who perhaps were unable to write their own name or pour a cup of coffee when they first moved in, regain their ability to do these basic practical tasks after we have worked with them. This does not include everyone, but we remain open for the possibility, encouraging their belief in themselves. Eventually, many of them regain their abilities. Marking the results on a graph enables an ongoing assessment of the individual's development and allows us to see which areas need reinforcing.

Screening the resident's abilities enables the staff to track any changes in a specific skill; for example, a resident may start slowing down when getting dressed. We note this as a focus area so that all staff will be mindful of training for this specific ability with this resident. Sometimes we see the resident regain an ability after having focused on it. At other times, our

---

[1] Kahle-Wrobleski, K., N. Coley, B. Lepage, C. Cantet, B. Vellas, S. Andrieu, PLASA/DSA Group. (2014). Understanding the complexities of functional ability in Alzheimer's disease: more than just basic and instrumental factors. Current Alzheimer Research, 11(4):357-366. DOI: 10.2174/156720501166614031710141419

[2] Galasko, D., Bennett, D., Sano, M., Ernesto, C., Thomas, R., Grundman, M., Ferris, S. (1997). An inventory to assess activities of daily living for clinical trials in Alzheimer's disease. The Alzheimer's Disease Cooperative Study. Alzheimer's Disease and Associated Disorders, 11 (Suppl. 2), S33-S39. PMID: 9236950.

observations tell us it is time to stop concentrating on it, as it will only make the resident more self-conscious about his or her declining condition.

In other words, the screening also tells us when to hold back—but only after we have thoroughly tried and assessed it. The last thing we want is for the staff to suddenly give up without any reason. It is sometimes hard to avoid this in a world where the staff are largely outnumbered by residents. Nevertheless, the screening system helps to raise our awareness. At the same time, it can be motivating for the staff to see the graph rising in connection to the resident's abilities. The typical curve shows a resident's abilities significantly improving soon after moving in, then remaining stable until the sudden dip before death.

The Norm:
"Physical therapy is usually on Tuesdays. . ."

When a new resident moves in at Dagmarsminde, he or she is not just burdened by a long list of medications, as discussed in Chapter 5. The resident also brings along the baggage of an inactive lifestyle. Maybe the person has been encouraged to sit back for years and has come to believe that he or she was too old and sick to move. Our job is to determine why a new resident is so passive. Is the person debilitated due to a disability that makes walking difficult or impossible? Does he or she suffer from dizziness? Or is there another reason for a sedentary state? Is it perhaps just a mental barrier? Has the person been stigmatized by caregiver assumptions about him or her? Self-doubt, which can be fed by well-meaning caregivers, could have shaped the person's identity and led to a distorted perception of his or her own abilities.

You have probably walked through the doors of a care home for people with dementia and noticed a jumble of wheelchairs and walkers parked to one side, and on the other side the residents slouching in the shared living room. Many nursing homes could be called "human parking lots." In these places, we do not see residents engaged in shared activities, especially not physical ones. If there is some form of exercise, then it usually happens once a week in a distant corner of the nursing home deemed suitable for exercising—perhaps a fitness room filled with machines, parallel walking bars, and giant balls. Everything is ready for when the physical therapist shows up; the staff would not think of doing exercises with the residents. It is not considered part of their skill set.

The underlying resistance to mobilizing the residents leads to another curiosity. Often, we see staff defending a resident's right to self-determination—typically in connection to the right to refuse the help the employee is supposed to offer. "We can't force the resident to exercise if he doesn't want to." And they do not. "We'll try next week; he didn't feel like it today." It is the staff's reluctance, and therefore not compassion, which supports the idea that a resident who does not feel like moving should not be made to. However, a resident is typically going to say, "No thank you," if exercise and training are not a part of the daily routine. The person may think, "Oh no, they're going to drag me over to that corner again. I can't take it. . . . It's better to say no." And the person has a right to say no in the name of self-determination. The staff member believes he or she is respecting the resident, and even feels proud enough of this to tell others in the office about it, thus reinforcing the notion.

Additionally, some people who work with older adults actually believe the people in their care are not capable of doing physical exercise. They may believe the older person has come to a standstill, is on a downward spiral, and is resigned to that state. In other words, isn't it just a fact of life that we all slowly fade away and die? It is true that the older we get, the less we can handle. But at the same time, the more physically fit we are, the more we stay active and the stronger we become. When most of a home's residents are kept medicated and inactive, washed in bed, and lifted to and from everything, then that home does not have confidence in the abilities of its staff or residents to safely engage in physical activities.

> With some practice, we begin to see each care situation as an opportunity to motivate the resident to move and to encourage ourselves to think more and more creatively.

In many places, the staff are afraid of getting too close—literally. They never even touch the residents. If using our hands is not an essential part of the care we provide, then we are not getting close enough to the resident for any training to happen. Once, I saw a particularly restless resident at a care home I was visiting. She just kept pacing the halls of the three buildings, which were connected by a garden courtyard in the middle. One day, I counted her going around 64 times. No one took the initiative to try to stop her. The staff stepped aside when she stormed past them and just let her walk and walk—lost, confused, in a cold sweat, and stressed. They figured her trance-like walk was part of her dementia. But it was not caused by her dementia. It continued to happen because no one stopped her or gave her something more stimulating to do instead. It never occurred to them that her surplus energy could be used for something more meaningful, such as taking a brisk walk outside, or doing some exercises, or even dancing with other people, all of which would develop her coordination and her awareness. Instead, all that untapped potential was wasted.

Objection:
"We're low-staffed, and we haven't had any training."

Exercise can be integrated into almost every part of care work. Regardless of education or experience, anyone can lead residents with dementia in physical activities. It does not take a certificate to use one's imagination. I am not suggesting that untrained staff members instruct residents in complicated physical therapy techniques. Obviously, professional skills are required for a disabled resident to sit up or even walk again. However, when a resident is not debilitated but only has become accustomed to not moving, a helpful care partner can encourage new ways of using the body while doing ordinary tasks. All it takes is common sense and a bit of imagination. I advise you to think creatively and plan how to squeeze in a few exercises as you go about your daily tasks with the residents. Encourage the resident, and always explain what you are doing.

No one needs a class to teach us how to move. We just do it. No course is going to teach us how to motivate and lead every individual resident. Every resident is different. Focusing on little exercises and introducing small movements into everyday life only requires that we consider who we are dealing with—consider the ability of the individual resident. For instance, letting the resident get up without help or walk from the living room to the bathroom does not necessarily take more time, but it can be immensely helpful to the person. With some practice, we begin to see each care situation as an opportunity to motivate the resident to move and to encourage ourselves to think more and more creatively.

Another benefit of this approach is that the more independent a resident becomes, the more time we create. If we go for a walk in the garden with a couple of the residents, they get some exercise, and in the meantime our colleagues can benefit from the extra free time. It will improve the day for everyone.

Summary

Policies and practices related to exercise and movement vary from home to home. However, whatever the culture of our own workplace, we can decide either to stay inactive and use our professional knowledge and skill set to come up with excuses for why there is not time for exercises, or to look for opportunities to move and enjoy spending time with the residents, bringing back joy and a sense of purpose to our work, as well as to their lives.

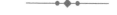

Questions for Reflection

1. Early in this chapter, the author describes having "expectations" of the residents, and how she and her staff use those expectations as a way of inspiring residents to keep moving. What do you think of the idea of having such expectations of people with dementia?

2. Consider the author's discussion of "self-determination" as it pertains to the right of the resident not to exercise if he or she does not feel like it. How do you weigh the resident's right to make decisions if you know that what you are encouraging them to do would be helpful to them?

3. Are there ideas or practices described in this chapter that you would like to see implemented in your own care home? What are the steps needed to make that happen? List any obstacles that you foresee, as well as people whose help you might enlist.

7

———◆◆———

Assistive Devices
for Mobility

So many assistive devices—medical equipment in all shapes and sizes designed to ease mobility—are used at nursing homes today that, at a glance, you would be forgiven for thinking, *Whoever lives here must be really sick.*

At Dagmarsminde, we shun elements that create a factory atmosphere, including these gadgets that often surround elders these days. The normal assumption is that these devices—especially wheelchairs, walkers, and lifts—exist to enable older people to become more independent. However, the exact opposite is usually true. Most of the assistive devices used by care staff the world over only add to the suffering of our elders by reinforcing disability and immobility and by discouraging both staff and residents from making any effort toward improvement. This is why I believe they should be shelved.

When I share my views in lectures to care home staff, I almost always hear an indignant sigh from a little group in the audience. Luckily, once they have heard my arguments, most of them walk away with at least a more critical stance toward assistive devices. I hope readers will think again before deciding to stay in the comfort of the familiar care world. In many places, including Denmark, care practice often revolves around the use of these devices. However, it doesn't have to be that way.

A Case Against Assistive Devices

Consider the general appearance of assistive devices for mobility. As soon as we remove them from the shared living space, the environment immediately feels more wholesome—more normal, less stigmatizing. When wheelchairs and other devices are placed throughout the shared spaces, they define the aesthetic of the room with their industrial shapes and their reminders of sickness and disability. Their presence loudly threatens our goal of a care home being a place where old people are cared for. Instead, we get the impression that the home is a kind of waiting room for death.

Many in our field have not considered how destructive these devices can be for the will to live. When we hide them, we immediately remove the overt signs of illness. This does not mean we pretend the residents are not older and do not have dementia. But there is no reason to saddle them with more illness or disability than they have. Our job is to enhance their lives so they feel as healthy as possible. We do not remove these devices just because they are an eyesore; aesthetically, their presence counteracts our professional perspective and our hopes for the residents. This aesthetic reason is only one part of our decision, though. The other is that when we remove the assistive devices, we ensure the residents *move more* and become a more active part of whatever is happening around them or to them. In short, the benefits of removing the wheelchairs and other devices from the environment usually outweigh any benefit of keeping them around.

Walkers

Sooner or later, walkers tend to appear in front of older adults, regardless of their abilities. They also tend to result in that hunched-over look, with residents staring at the ground instead of keeping their eyes on the world in front of them. Almost everyone using a walker has bad posture as they inch their way forward. It is hard to resist the urge to walk over and help them straighten up. But we are not the only ones who feel that way; it clearly frustrates the residents, too. Looking at them, we notice how many of them look tense or stressed as they push their walkers around.

Our job is to shoulder the weight of the world for our residents, to offer them a life rich with experience, and to help stoke their curiosity. However, it is hard to be curious with a view that is limited to a 90-degree angle. Why curb the resident's perception even more than dementia already has? Consider how the walker can make the resident feel when constantly bound to a device. It is our task to help our residents regain self-confidence. Walking upright means walking with confidence.

A walker constantly gets in the way when you try to move around, creating an obstacle for the resident trying to pass between pieces of furniture or walk in and out of rooms. Also, residents with dementia often do not use their walkers properly. When they stumble, the walker rolls off without them. Their pace can become forced and unnatural when hurried on wheels.

But what do we do with the walkers? Should we just sneak in one night and carry them off? Not exactly. The ability to move without a walker varies from person to person. For some residents, it will feel perfectly natural to allow a staff member to hold their hand or support them with an arm under their shoulder; in cases like these, the walker can be removed immediately. For others, we need to develop a detailed plan for gradually helping the resident feel safe without the walker. Thus, we replace the walker with *company*. Only another human being can adequately follow the resident's movements and sense when he or she needs support.

It is important to note that removing the walker usually goes hand in hand with tapering the medicine. By increasing a resident's strength, we naturally improve his or her balance. Making this change is as much about removing the stigma of a walker from the resident as it is about creating a sense of confidence. In my experience, when we take away the walker, 9 out of 10 residents do fine without it. For some, however, they have depended on it for so many years that they get very uncomfortable if we take it away, so we keep using it.

> *When you take away the walker, the staff*
> *automatically feel closer to the resident.*

My point is that we should not automatically assume everyone will feel uncomfortable when we remove the walker. In reality, very few of them do. I often recall how many older people used a cane in the past. It was a symbol of old age. Today, the walker is more widely used. In addition to being a lot less elegant than a cane, a walker discourages upright, independent movement. The walker is partly to blame for reducing the individual to a kind of stereotype of old age and illness.

Here, it is important to emphasize how critical it is to have enough staff members available to help and support a resident who is learning to walk without a walker. This does not mean having one employee per resident. We usually have three staff members working with 12 residents. Most importantly, think solidarity. When you take away the walker, the staff automatically feel closer to the resident.

Wheelchairs

Ironically, someone sitting in a regular chair is a lot more mobile than if he or she is sitting in a wheelchair. People can become completely paralyzed in a wheelchair. It is harder to move your arms and legs, and you are practically stuck there. This is one of the main reasons we take the residents out of the wheelchairs and have them sit in normal chairs. If they cannot walk, we push their wheelchair into the shared living room and then help them into one of the chairs. If a resident needs support in order to sit upright, then we choose a chair with an armrest. It takes a bit of trial and error.

Moving a wheelchair user to a regular chair can be a fantastic experience. The resident becomes a whole new person. It is easier to see the true individual as he or she was before developing dementia, back before anything had changed, when the person went on vacations and joined in family gatherings. It is as if the resident suddenly spreads his or her wings, revealing personality and wonderful charisma. Maybe the person leans forward, places a hand on the table, and crosses his or her legs. This is how the person used to sit, with his or her guard let down; it feels natural to look around and participate. When this happens, there is no question that we have done the resident a favor by helping him or her out of the wheelchair. The person's mind has been put at ease as well as the body. That is the beautiful and magical part about helping residents from their wheelchair into an ordinary piece of furniture.

Another benefit is that the act of moving from a wheelchair to the ordinary chair is an exercise in itself. The resident has to stand up, turn around, and move in a way he or she would not be able to when sitting in the wheelchair all day. Needless to say, the staff help with the move. Sometimes the move might require two staff members. Because the employees in our care culture agree that people should not sit in a wheelchair all day long, they are willing to support the residents as they attempt the move.

Life at Our Home

A new resident arrived in a giant wheelchair along with instructions to transfer her with a lift at all times. When we asked her why she needed a wheelchair, she wasn't actually sure. We asked, "Should we try to see if you can get up and take a couple of steps?" We didn't get a chance to hear her response before she was up and walking. She paced around her room. We had to move the furniture out of the way so she didn't walk into chairs and tables. Finally, we had to ask her to sit down again. In time she learned to navigate safely without our help. She also learned to climb stairs again.

Of course, some residents will never regain the ability to sit in an ordinary chair. Those who are partially disabled or extremely stiff from Parkinson's disease, for instance, will have to continue to use the wheelchair. Additionally, a person with permanent sensory damage may repeatedly fall forward out of an ordinary chair. These are the exceptions that require the help of special wheelchairs.

It is also important to state that wheelchairs that are not in use in between the residents' moves should not be left standing in the hallways or even be visible in the shared living spaces. We place them out of sight when they are not in use, rolled away into the resident's room. They should never be a part of the everyday view of the residents. Although the wheelchairs are out of the picture, they are always available when needed to help residents move from one place to another. For example, if we move a resident sitting at the dining table out to the terrace, then we fetch the wheelchair for support and move the person into one of the garden chairs. When it is time for our daily exercises, we fetch the wheelchair again and bring the person over to one of our chairs placed in a circle for the exercise activity. At this point, the resident is already somewhat warmed up, having performed the "exercise" of getting up out of the wheelchair and sitting down in a chair.

Lifts

We believe staff should try to minimize the use of lifts, or hoists. We rarely use them. In general, they are only necessary during the final weeks of a resident's life, when the person no longer comprehends the moving process or lacks the strength to stand without help. In these cases, using the lift is the most low-impact choice for the resident.

It is possible to move weakened people without lifts as long as there are at least one or two staff members trained in lift-independent techniques. When we shift our focus from the assistive device and the many ways it can be used, what we are left with is the strength and maneuverability of one's own body.

The staff member and the resident collaborate—you could even call it a kind of dance, in which the resident leads. The goal is establishing a flow in which the resident's and staff's movements merge during the process. Consider the center of balance: Where is it? We try to find the most natural way for the resident to get up, and we see if the person's weak points can be adequately supported by the staff's body. We try to transfer our momentum to the resident. We use this method throughout, right up until the resident reaches the final phase of the disease.

If the assistive devices are present, the staff will use them. If the assistive devices are gone, the staff will find another way.

Rethinking Transfer

When we decide to go down the device-independent path, it is important we remain open to reconsidering how to transfer the residents. We have to recognize and acknowledge that there are always other possibilities. If we are unsure about any part of our technique, then we need to admit it and talk about where and why we are uncertain. In this way, we can find a better, more sound solution.

Lifts are generally a "no go" at Dagmarsminde. I strongly recommend that architects focus on the more inspiring features when designing the interior of care homes. They should not plan for a lift in the ceiling of every room, where, as in a slaughterhouse, the staff can hoist up the old bodies and swing them across the room. It is basic human psychology: If the assistive devices are present, the staff will use them. If the assistive devices are gone, the staff will find another way. If a lift is absolutely necessary, then the team thoroughly assesses the situation before putting it into use. There will always be some employees who advocate the use of the lift. But by and large, they need some very strong arguments before I will even consider it.

I have covered the most common—and for the residents, often intrusive—assistive devices. But I recommend considering other devices as well. Whenever a situation seems to call for an assistive device, stop to consider if there is an alternative. The indiscriminate use of these devices transforms caregiving into something mechanical you just need to get through, and this mentality is to the detriment of the residents in your care.

The Norm:
Who Is Assisted by Assistive Devices?

Many care homes look like factories. The ceilings are lined with tracks for motorized lifts. The residents sit around in wheelchairs, where the visitor mainly sees the back of the chair or the raised leg rests. The wheelchairs are also often reclined, so the residents spend much of their time half-lying down.

A lot of effort goes into developing high-tech devices with all sorts of functions that can be adjusted with merely a click. Care homes buy the best that technology has to offer. But these assistive devices are not usually installed for the sake of the residents. The huge investment in lifts and multifunctional wheelchairs is mainly implemented for work and safety reasons—in order to make it easier for the staff to be at work and to safeguard the facility against lawsuits. Once again, the fear-mongering mentality overrules. Dealing with older adults is apparently dangerous.

The way people refer to their work at care homes today makes it sound like risky business. Explained to an outsider, it almost sounds as though care home employees are working with dangerous chemicals or being sent into combat. Of course, as everyone in the staff office or the county agrees, the job *certainly* is dangerous, so we had better install some devices to make it safer for the staff. *Voila!* Wheelchairs and walkers for everyone. In one easy solution, all the different challenges faced by individual residents are solved and the work environment is made "safe and sound."

In some places, such as Denmark, unions dictate what we have to do in order to take care of the employees. The idea is that employees have a right not to be exposed to any kind of danger, so they should approach any physical interactions with residents only with great caution. In other places, policies mandating the use of lifts and other devices exist to protect the organization from lawsuits or other consequences in the event of an accident involving injury to a resident or employee. Whatever the reason for the mandates, though, they ignore the fact that the care home exists to take care of people who are no longer able to care for themselves. Staff are not hired, and care homes do not exist, to be fearful. The prevailing attitude means that the weakest ones—the residents—will have to fend for themselves in the name of staff health and safety and the protection of the home from any liability.

The staff at many ordinary care homes are instructed not to try to catch a resident who stumbles; they must step back and let the resident fall. And, when the person is lying on the ground, the employee should not help him up or even touch him. It is a *no-hands* policy. The only permitted way to help is with a lift. Lifts and other devices are always accompanied by protocols—they offer a so-called solution to every situation. Huge amounts of money are invested to install ceiling hoists in every corner. Anywhere in the care home, a staff member can quickly snap a carabiner on a resident, thereby watching the person grow weaker instead of more self-reliant and stronger. Although lifts may seem to help employees and care homes, they diminish the residents' identity, eliminating their most essential connection to themselves as human beings.

In some places, care home residents are not even allowed to go to the bathroom by themselves. The staff think it is easier and faster for residents to use the lift. Bathroom visits are expedited by wheeling the resident to his or her own room and hoisting him or her up and over to the bed. The resident lands on top of a clean incontinence pad, the full pad is removed, and the resident is lifted right back into the wheelchair. I am not sure why this procedure has become so common. If a lift has to be used, it could be used to help the resident actually sit on the toilet and urinate. This only further demonstrates how wide-spread use of the device diminishes empathy and compassion for older people—not to mention the ability to care for themselves.

These examples demonstrate how the field of nursing is prostrating itself to technology. We are surrounded by gadgets. We even have beds that automatically turn the residents. You push a button and—*presto!*—the resident faces the other way; there are no more long conversations to convince the resident he or she can still turn without help.

The excessive and inappropriate use of assistive devices is especially harmful because it usually happens too early in the course of the disease. No one pays attention to this injustice as long as the real goal is to check a box with the least amount of physical strain or to comply with county or organizational regu-lations. Employees get accustomed to working in this kind of mechanical environment and can forget to think critically about it. After a while, this way of providing care can feel comfortable and safe. The few who actually question it are ignored or worse and give up, realizing that their questions are not appreciated.

From time to time, employees can be injured when working at a care home. As nurses, we have chosen to work with the sick and weak. It is a job that requires a certain amount of physical labor. We have to be strong. Yet, although the work is obviously strenuous at times, staff are often told not to move a finger—or, anyway, not to use any of their upper body strength. I have seen staff afraid of physical contact—both of being touched and of touching others. They automatically assume a lift or wheel-chair must be used with residents. The device comes before the human being. The work becomes short-sighted. It is a pity, because this mentality prevents the employees from ever expe-riencing the thrill of doing things differently.

Objection:
"We have a lot of work years ahead of us."

A common argument for the use of assistive devices is that it protects the staff members from injury, which could cause them to have to leave the care sector. However, whether and how long we stay in care work depends a great deal on our inspiration. Developing ourselves while caring for others offers motivation to continue. We grow when we are able to brainstorm with colleagues in order to find new solutions no one thought possible, such as new ways to help a resident out of bed and to the bathroom without causing injury to ourselves. A factory environment is diametrically opposed to this kind of activity, and it can be a demotivating and alienating situation in which to work. It is fixed, without variation or possibility for interaction. Care work becomes an automatic, mechanical act. Nursing loses its meaning. The staff need to feel their work has purpose, that they have something to offer and can improve the lives of the people living at the care home. If they are always walking around doing the same automatic tasks in the same way, day in and day out, it is no surprise if they lose interest in staying. That kind of environment can be draining for the body, mind, and spirit. I believe staff retention improves when people find the work pleasurable and inspiring. Assistive devices do not inspire anyone.

Summary

Rather than easing the workload or making anyone safer, assistive devices only make working with the residents more cumbersome. If the residents are constantly immobilized, they get heavier and more difficult to work with. They stop cooperating. They give up and accept their role as "dead weight." Believing that these devices are helpful or even necessary all the time is a misconception born from never having seen what happens when they are put away. People are encouraged to mechanically carry out their tasks, as if at an industrial slaughterhouse. But we work in a care home, not a factory. Assistive devices are predominately a symbol of a world that has distanced itself from the very people they were meant to help. The vulnerable people in our care have basic human needs, which devices cannot begin to fulfill. Next time you think you need to use an assistive device, see if there is another way to meet that need.

------◆◆◆------

Questions for Reflection

1. Do you find the vision of a care home without ready assistive devices appealing? What are some of the challenges you see with that approach, and what are some ways of overcoming them?

2. Do you agree with the author's view that assistive devices "add to the suffering of our elders by reinforcing disability and immobility"? Explain your reasoning.

3. What is your organization's policy on the use of assistive devices? Are you happy with that policy, and if not, how might it be changed?

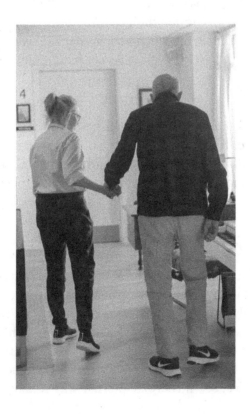

8

⸺ ◆ ⸺

Working with Energies

A Dynamic Balance

DEMENTIA CREATES INNER CHAOS. IN this chapter, I explain how we restore and maintain balance by treating the care home as a sacred place. A balanced care home is one in which the staff are conscious of heavy and light energies. By "energies," I mean natural life forces, of which we are part and parcel—life forces transferred from nature to people, from people to nature, and from person to person. The residents at a care home—as well as the staff—are affected by these energies, which they also help to generate and share.

First and foremost, we have a circular understanding of a care home, in which we are each a part of a greater whole. To put it plainly, we cannot separate our understanding of a resident from the changing seasons, growth in the garden, the flower in the vase, the cat in the armchair, or the person next to us at the dinner table. A holistic approach to care work extends beyond the individual. Everything has an influence on everything else. In some sense, the care home is like a giant organism, which we work to preserve in its entirety.

Working with this mindset means first acknowledging that the natural world around us has a consciousness—not just human beings. This idea seems self-evident if everything is seen as connected, and yet it can seem almost superstitious to say that nature has a consciousness. It is easier to relate to this idea, for example, if you think about a flower turning to face the sun. This kind of dynamic, sensory experience is perfectly normal to us as humans. We are part of nature, and nature is part of us.

If you are still finding it difficult to say out loud that the tree, the earth, and the stone have a consciousness, then consider this: Our commercialized, mechanized, and evidence-based society has led us to believe that our intelligence is exceptional, on account of our abilities to rationalize, analyze, and systematize a mountain of information. Our focus on these rational abilities gives them primacy in our society, and we therefore have a bias toward rational experiences.

But we also exist on another level of consciousness that includes, for example, dreaming, falling in love, or playing sports. These experiences involve a level of "thinking" that is not rational. It allows us to be carried by a more irrational and self-regulating, natural universe. The rational person would call this level of existence the "unconscious," or perhaps "a belief in something larger than ourselves." If we see these experiences and our openness to them as another set of colors on our palette that we may commonly overlook, then another world opens up for valuing and acknowledging other forms of consciousness. It becomes clearer how we as people—precisely like the flower—have a sensory consciousness and therefore do not need to feel removed from nature, but rather can open ourselves to be part of its dynamic. Care workers, especially those who work with people living with dementia, are at their best when they are open to this unconscious energy of life.

The Spiritual Care Home

We experience these energies on a daily basis with our residents, in connection with this less rational way of approaching the world. This sensory dimension is fundamental for our care work because the residents, due to their dementia, often find themselves in an irrational state—perhaps in that same consciousness I just referred to—which those of us without dementia do not always acknowledge. At the same time, they are not always able to access that rational and more neutral consciousness necessary for maintaining a balanced mind. That is where we come in.

We encourage our staff members to help our residents stay in balance between "our" rationality and their understanding of reality. This demands that the staff member respect the resident's consciousness but at the same time maintain a level of rational thinking within that communication. For instance, a woman whose husband is long dead asks, "When is my husband coming to visit?" Depending on the needs of the individual, the staff member might say, "I understand that you want to see your husband, but let me ask you, as I'm not sure: Do you think he is still alive?" If the resident says yes, the staff member could, in a caring way, explain that her husband is no longer alive, and that she is now living here at the nursing home so that she is not alone, can be taken care of, and gets help when she needs it.

In many instances, presenting this new, rational narrative in a kind and caring way makes sense to the resident, who then feels respected and in touch with the rational world. This approach works when the staff member can talk rationally with the resident. Sometimes, however, the resident talks in his or her own language—what we might call "nonsense" or "gibberish." In a moment like this, it is very important for the staff member to be able to enter into his or her own nonrational consciousness and imagination to answer and talk "normally," responding to the nonrational language as if it is normal. What is important is helping the resident to *feel* a sense of rationality in the dialogue.

Balance should not be understood as a state of equilibrium. The goal is not to achieve a fixed state of calm and comfort because, in fact, that is not a natural state. We try to work toward a more dynamic type of balance, where the aim is to prevent stagnation. For instance, a resident experiencing gloom and anger should be allowed to express these feelings, but we need to be there to support the person during this episode. Residents can get stuck in their dreamy, fluid consciousness, and we have to help them improve their mental flexibility by stimulating healthy fluctuations. If a resident gets stuck in a moody state, we strive to help them toward the possibility of a different outlook—one of courage, for example, or hope. This is not a state of equilibrium, with no strong feelings or experiences. We need to allow for natural ripples. We adopt the attitude, for example, that a new challenging behavior is a form of communication that confronts our views and refines our decision-making abilities, ultimately leading us toward a strategy that will improve the resident's life.

Working with Energies

Our care work, even more than we might realize from our studies or training, should draw upon a spiritual dimension geared to finding harmony with nature and, by extension, our residents. I am not talking about "spiritual" in any religious sense, or even as *good* or *bad* energies.

When we talk about energies, we label them *heavy* or *light* instead of good or bad. If we related to energies as good or bad (positive or negative), our judgment could hinder our ability to help. Words such as heavy and light, however, allow for interpretation and change. We view stagnation—a fixed energy—as a threat to our care work. A light energy is clear and straightforward, and it brightens up a room as it brightens up our day. We feel at home, secure, and confident that a situation is stable. A heavy energy gives us that dreaded feeling that something is uncertain or seems "lost," which can put us on our guard and make us feel uneasy. Chaos is rooted in heavy energies.

A waterfall of energy pouring out of a ranting resident could be considered light if it helps the resident restore his or her inner calm. It is a kind of natural reaction that offers temporary relief, just as a walk on the beach in the rain may offer relief.

This understanding of energy is not about there being one way to be. Rather, we are encouraged to sense when an energy is in dynamic balance—at one with nature. Energy can feel light, of course, during nice, quiet conversations, or when we are happy and smiling, but it can sometimes also get outright jumpy within a dynamic balance. Think about riding a bike and being able to smoothly pedal forward without thinking about fluctuations on the ground or the varying movements of the body.

> *Energies are everything we cannot account for with guidelines, task lists, methods, or manuals.*

We have all felt a surge of irrational thoughts in our lives before; in fact, they are often part of our decision making. Imagine you are looking for a new place to live and you know which street you want to live on. You are standing on that street looking at two houses that are both for sale. Both houses meet your needs for greenery and all the physical and spatial requirements. At first glance, they look equally well-kept and pretty, and they are the same price. However, one of the houses appeals to you more than the other. It seems cozy. It feels good just to look at it. You sense it has a good atmosphere, that it is a place you could call home. When you look at the other house, you might get a sinking feeling, as if it were teetering on a cliff. This subtle sense makes you feel unwelcome. The house shuts itself off to you, feels oppressive; you don't even feel like going inside.

Energies are everything we cannot account for with guidelines, task lists, methods, or manuals. On the other hand, since we are a part of these energies ourselves and can direct our attention accordingly, we can help transform a heavy energy into a light one. An excess of unmanaged heavy energies can be destructive to a care home. Neither the staff nor the residents benefit from too much heavy energy. People with dementia, in particular, react if the mood gets too heavy. They might have lost their normal capabilities, but they are very sensitive and react to anything that might weigh them down—or lift their spirits. The rest of us might not always pick up on these energies as we busily impose our thoughts on the world around us. The residents live in a world of extreme sensing, one that staff who are stuck in a rational mindset cannot always perceive. It is important, then, to fine-tune our ability to perceive, understand, and—when needed—work to adjust the energy at our care home.

A heavy energy can feel like an oppressive, wet fog that increases gradually so that we barely notice it at first. It may seem that things are going well. The residents are tended to, the place looks neat and tidy, and we have set some goals and have almost achieved them. The residents seem calm and quiet. Maybe they have just had a good sing-along—but we might sense something is not right. There is a lingering unease, and it could cause us to want to give up—or face it.

Heavy energies can arise, for example, in the unspoken exchanges between residents and staff members. The source could be something from a resident's past, or it could be the staff member themselves, whose lack of integrity feels disruptive in the room. There could be a third, unknown external factor. We have to remove the wall that exists within heavy energies in order for our acts of care to be meaningful. That is why it is essential to understand these energies.

Heavy energies are always connected to fear. An atmosphere of heavy energy often presides over care homes that focus on what is difficult or irretrievable in the resident's condition. Care staff who do not focus on the person's remaining strengths and abilities, who do not encourage them to continue to grow and enjoy life, propagate heavy energies.

Light energies are generally easier to pick up on because they spread joy and ease to everyone in a room. Often, they arise as a natural reaction after the heavy energies have been removed. However, it is important to remember that light energies naturally occur if we do not work against them.

The point of this chapter is that we have a *choice*. We can make a conscious effort to redirect heavy energies into

Life at Our Home

At one point, the room of one of our residents had a heavy energy. We talked a lot about how hard it was to make the room light again when we were with her. We thought we were doing everything right. We gave ourselves plenty of time with the resident in the morning. She smiled and wanted to give us a hug as soon as she opened her eyes. Yet there was still something strange about her room. When two of the staff were in there, we almost always got irritated at each other. We brought it up, and tried leaving the room and coming back, first together and then alone. Then we went back in, sat down, and simply let our senses absorb the room.

My nurse colleague Lotte, who is known for her spiritual approach to nursing, thought she sensed some unresolved issues within the family that we had not heard about. Perhaps it was an unpleasant incident, which must have led to what she described as shaming.

Regardless of whether Lotte was right about someone in the family having been shamed, her reaction gave us an incentive to make some little changes to lighten the energy in her room. We decided to add or do something to the room, which would help lighten the energy. We did not move any of her personal belongings, but we began stopping by her room more often to look at pictures from her youth and pictures of her family as well. You might say that we went out of our way to work with her fear of whatever it was that had happened. Meanwhile, we also overcame our own fear of being in the room, and the heavy energy left.

After our experience with the room, we went on a trip to the woods. We usually do this anyway, but this time we had the goal of putting an end to any lingering heavy energy. We asked a couple of the residents to find some objects they liked, and one of the women found a beautiful branch with some pretty white mushrooms growing on it. Wrapping her arms around the yard-and-a-half–long stick, she let us know she was determined to keep it. We lay it across the back of the wheelchair, brought it home, and placed it in a big vase in the middle of the living room. It became both a turning point and our main topic of conversation— the residents couldn't keep their eyes off the pretty mushrooms. The branch helped us create a light atmosphere again.

light ones. We cannot completely eliminate heavy energies, of course. We would not want to, anyway, because they make us yearn for the opposite. They motivate us to let in the light.

The ability to perceive energies runs parallel with other virtues I have mentioned, especially good judgment. We can only transform the heavy to light by understanding our own responsibility and role in connection to them. Once we have opened ourselves to this kind of sensing, it becomes fairly uncomplicated. One could say that this sensory perception is the first and most natural skill that care workers have developed. As human beings, we have an innate capacity for it.

When we are trying to figure out the reason for the heavy energy, the ability to make sense of what we perceive is fundamental. It is not a question of being right or wrong, but rather of identifying the reason for the heavy energy and acknowledging our part in it. Then we have to try to turn it around and make it light again.

At Dagmarsminde, we often use our natural surroundings as a way of connecting to the bigger picture. We create a sense of wholeness by drawing from the light and bright energies of nature. Acknowledging a soul and sensory existence of everything—the air, the sea, the animals, even the wooden floors we walk on—generates respect. The holistic, circular nature of our thinking leads to an understanding that we are constantly part of *what is* and *what has been*.

Likewise, I believe that those of us working at care homes need to acknowledge that these homes have souls and are subject to changes in energies as much as human beings are. Nursing is more than just facts and reason, and it is crucial that we respect that. Nursing involves everything we believe in plus tuning into the in-between—the fleeting silences that are always there. We are not psychics, but we take our intuitive senses seriously. It takes practice to learn to trust in these instincts.

If we notice a heavy energy, to a greater or lesser degree, we pay attention to it, and then try to counter it with something light. This could be as seemingly insignificant as moving around some pictures in the windowsill—maybe taking one away—or bringing a branch or flowers inside from the woods; nature works wonders in our work. It could also be something as simple as changing a seating arrangement. Some groups of people create a heavy energy together, not necessarily because of dementia or their personalities. When we shake things up a little, we can facilitate change for the better. For example, we might sense that things will have to be done in a certain way on this particular day to meet a resident's care situation. This is not something that we read about or will ever read in a text-book, but we can feel deep inside that right now we need to slow down and do things a little differently.

Working within these instinctual energies implies a sacred-ness, a necessary acknowledgment that something greater than ourselves and what we are doing exists. This connection, which some might call a sixth sense, in reality is connected to all of our senses. In our logic-driven minds, however, it is easy to dis-miss the spiritual dimension of the world we live in.

Seeing the world through this lens does not mean walk-ing around intoxicated by the supernatural. We are not joined by mystical spirits flying around the room. We simply learn to discern energies, and then we take responsibility for changing them if they are too heavy. The light energies must be rekin-dled in people again. As we develop our sensitivity and judg-ment, these adjustments follow automatically. Our presence brightens the room and our residents feel it too.

Stop, look, and listen. Connect to something greater, to nature and to the universe. Take the example of the resident who has her own indecipherable language that she speaks in. She does not need to be corrected, only heard and acknowledged. Her lan-guage does not need to be explained and understood, or necessar-ily even "fixed" by figuring out a way to stop it. We acknowledge that it is merely part of the bigger picture. The staff member is not just pulling the strings at the care home, but rather is work-ing with energies, sharpening his or her perception, and acting accordingly—eventually becoming better at restoring balance.

As noted earlier, touch is part of the care we provide at Dagmarsminde. We are not "hands-off" when it comes to our residents. When we touch or embrace a resident in our care, we can absorb the person's heavy energies, and in return send them our light energy. Later, during a walk in the woods, when we lean up against a tree, we can transfer those absorbing, heavy energies through its bark. The tree becomes our inspiration to take the hands of a resident and guide him or her down the winding path through the forest, leaving the tree behind us to send those heavy energies down to its roots, and further into the earth, from where they may sprout, continuing the natural cycle of energy.

There is nothing strange about searching our feelings and trying to create a dynamic balance. It is only natural, another way of understanding the world, a way practiced by people across the globe long before technology and pharmaceuticals were developed. Sometimes, not much effort is required. At other times, we have to make a radical change and struggle to restore the light energy. But once it is restored, there is no doubt about it. Whenever that happens at Dagmarsminde, I feel the place get stronger.

The Norm:
Nothing Is Sacred

Most care homes today do not pay attention to spiritual values. Let's say you go visit your father, who lives on the second floor of a care home. As soon as you enter the building, you bump into that same 100-year-old man who is always pushing himself around in his wheelchair asking for help. A group of women sit at the communal dining table, each in her own wheelchair, silent, head hanging. A little farther down the hall, you pass a resident whose pants are falling down. You hear a loud, obnoxious voice from inside the kitchen: "What about you, Pernille? You off this weekend?" The staff are hidden behind a big "No Entry" sign, which really means "No Residents." The implication is that the residents are not desirable company.

After you have collected your father in his room and rolled him over to the elevator, you hold your breath because of the strong smell of urine. The elevator doors slide open, and your path is blocked by a staff member who shouts: "Look who's getting a walk today . . . What do you say, Mr. Hansen, wanna go outside?" The buddy-buddy tone is an attempt to demonstrate familiarity between the staff and resident, but it oozes with indifference, as if the staff member has been instructed to be "chummy" with the relatives—one of many tasks to check off on the to-do list.

This example illustrates what happens in many care homes, where staff do not feel as if they are part of anything sacred. They are at work because they *have* to be. Yet when we do not feel ourselves to be part of something greater, our work can become meaningless. When we feel as if nothing we do makes a difference, it influences the way we act. The ambience degrades, which affects the behavior of both residents and staff. The care home becomes a prison or junkyard with no code of conduct. Staff members talk loudly without regard for the people who live there, roll their eyes with their colleagues when a resident is having difficulties, or enter a resident's room without knocking. Even death is not sacred in a place like this. When a resident is dying, an older staff member might shout to the new temp, "If you haven't seen a death before, come on in and watch."

But a care home is and should always be a sacred place. Sacred spaces require discretion. Think what would happen to your experience of a care home if you entered with respect and humility, lowering your voice and walking quietly—not out of fear, but out of the deepest consideration, even veneration, for the people there. It might be comparable to the feeling of entering a house where you have been invited for dinner for the first time. You would want to be extra polite and respectful of the home and the people who have invited you.

When I give talks, I sometimes encounter a reluctance to see care homes as sacred, especially among the more hardened individuals in the audience who have worked in care homes for many years. "Give me a break, it's just a living room," they say. They are wrong, though. A living room in a care home is not just some place people randomly gather. It is a dynamic space in which we share an experience. We can either sanctify the place and each other with what we bring to our interactions and maintain balance, or we can leave the place feeling gloomy and dead. The choice is ours.

This approach is about letting in the light, both physically and spiritually. It is about paying attention to what it means to be human. Energies are all around us, and also within us. They are not separate from us. That is why we are capable of creating change. We are responsible for perceiving, considering, and becoming aware of the energies. Stated differently, we are either a part of the problem or a part of the solution. The quality of the care at a nursing home improves when we sharpen our senses and become aware of the world around us. That is when the quality of caring is brought to another level.

I once visited a dementia unit that seemed on the verge of collapse; no one there was happy. The staff themselves had an unhealthy, pallid look, and the atmosphere was about as respectful as an appliance store on Black Friday. Then one day, one of the staff members, listening to her inner voice, suddenly got up on a chair and hung a branch from the ceiling with yellow Easter eggs. In the middle of all the heaviness, everyone was drawn to the branch. Residents talked about it and admired it. The little branch suddenly became a sign of hope.

Objection:
"Hocus-pocus doesn't change the fact we're understaffed."

I have heard many arguments that dismiss the kind of spiritual approach I have described. Admittedly, it can be difficult to grasp. It is not a set of tasks that can be implemented with a list. Paying attention to energies, however, is not about having enough time or staff. Energies are universal and therefore transcend time. Becoming aware that we are part of something greater is not about staffing. Of course, when we are busy running up and down the halls, it can be hard to tune in to the heavy energy. Having to run around generates a heavy energy in itself. Maybe we are struggling with budget cuts or colleagues on sick leave, and it feels as if it is all on our shoulders. In those moments, it is up to us to check in with our feelings and notice what is happening around us, and around our residents. Do we give up and run away? Do we get scared? We have to remain aware of the heavy energy in order for it to lessen. It might not happen immediately, but once we understand our own part in it, we can start to counter it.

With practice, working with an awareness of energy can become second nature—an integral part of our work. When you are just learning, it might take more than a day or two, but soon you will brighten any room you enter, and you will have a positive influence on the people in your care as well as on those around you. Increasing your awareness of energies, and working with them, will help you even if you feel overworked.

Even a short-staffed home or unit will benefit from care staff who try to pay attention to energies in their daily work. This approach can improve individual care and end what I call the dark spiral. It starts with a home on a tight schedule. The environment is chaotic and the staff members lose track of what is happening. The chaos affects the residents, they take a turn for the worse, the schedule gets even tighter, and so on. With awareness of heavy energies, the staff of the home or unit could be busy, but then someone might ask why they are so busy and consider how he or she might inspire the residents. Later, the person could reflect on whether things have improved. It is an exercise in self-reflection. One action may not necessarily solve the problem, but if all staff work with this mindset—especially with encouragement from leadership—things will get better. An increased awareness can help save the day.

Here is an example to consider: You are running down the hall with your arms full of trash bags and dirty laundry.

Imagine a resident comes stumbling down the hall and you sense them trying to make eye contact. Ordinarily you might look down, avoiding the resident's eyes, because you are busy and do not feel you can stop. What would happen if, instead, you looked the resident in the eye, and said, "Hi, I want to talk to you, but first I have to get rid of these bags. Okay?" This is an honest response because, despite the tight schedule, you recognize what is sacred.

Summary

We all are a part of the grand scheme of things, and each of us has an effect on the people around us, especially on those with dementia. We pass on heavy energies or light energies. We either strive to make life better for our residents or they are simply part of our job. Spiritual energy is in the words you are reading, your mindset, what you tell others, your body language, and your actions after you put down this book. Try approaching the people in your care with this awareness if you are not already doing so, and see what happens.

———— • ◆ • ————

Questions for Reflection

1. Do you relate to the author's description of a spiritual, energetic, or sacred aspect to care work? Try to describe the experience from your own perspective or understanding.

2. Have you experienced the feeling of knowing instinctively what needed to be done in a caring situation even though it was not part of your training or even understanding? What happened? And how has it affected your care work since?

3. Take a moment to pause in your own workplace. Tune in to the energy or sacredness of the situation, as you understand it. How does this level of attention affect, or not, your experience of the situation and what you are able to bring to it?

9

·◆·

The Circadian Rhythm

Open-eyed Residents

THE LAST THING WE WANT to see at our care home is a group of sleepy residents, snoozing away the day. On the contrary, we want to see them sleeping through the night and alert during the day, responsive to the world around them. In order to have open-eyed residents, we have to keep track of when they need to rest.

We begin by following their circadian rhythm: We stimulate the residents as much as we can during waking hours, and allow them to recoup mentally through sleep, so they are ready for more experiences upon waking. Our residents do not take sleeping pills (once tapered off), and much of the focus is on their natural daily rhythm, but the mindset and approach I present here are also relevant for those who are still on medication.

The need to understand a resident's sleep patterns is often underestimated in the care sector, but this understanding is essential for enabling care work. At Dagmarsminde, we observe the residents on a daily basis and talk to each other when we have noticed an individual getting tired. We explore the situation in detail, including the following:

- How we can tell the person is tired
- How the person has been sleeping at night

- Wakeup times
- Times of day when we have observed tiredness

Slowly, but surely, we start to understand the resident's rhythm.

When residents with dementia are active during the day, they tire more quickly in the evening. Over time, as their dementia advances, residents need increasing amounts of sleep. In general, most need about 11–13 hours of sleep during the night and a good long nap of 1–2 hours during the day. When a resident enters a more advanced phase of the illness, what I call the *weakening phase*, he or she will need around 16–18 hours of sleep, with the main segment of it lasting from early evening to morning. I will focus more on the weakening phase in Part Two of this book, but as long as the resident is within the more stable rehabilitating phase, there is plenty of opportunity to establish a circadian rhythm that allows for days filled with meaningful activity.

The residents are at their best in the morning after a good night's sleep. When they wake, they are confident and coordinated in their movements, speech, comprehension, perception of reality, and ability to hold a conversation. Importantly, they are also the most positive at this time about participating in the day's activities. In the early hours, they are eager to seize the day.

As the day proceeds, most will need a little extra sleep. Residents who have been up since early daylight, around 6:00 a.m., are likely to need a rest by 8:00 or 9:00 a.m. Spending a long time in the warm-water therapy pool, followed by socializing at the breakfast table, quickly tires the early risers. A resident might start slouching or repeatedly standing up and sitting down. Or, we might notice the person putting his or her glass down inside a cup or trying to reorganize the place setting of someone who is still eating breakfast.

These examples illustrate how the need for sleep can suddenly creep up on the resident. It is important for the staff member to take action immediately. The resident needs to be led away for a rest, before becoming more exhausted, which can lead to restlessness. This is part of the balancing act. The staff member approaches the resident and picks up his or her plate and glass, adding, "It looks as if you've finished eating." Then the staff member offers to show the resident a nice comfortable place to lie down and relax. She walks alongside the resident to the resting area, where the person is calmly and lovingly supported while lying down. The staff member asks, "Can I take off your glasses? I'll put them right over here." If the resident nods yes, the staff member removes the glasses; the same goes for the resident's shoes. Then the staff member arranges and tucks a blanket around the tired resident.

The above is not a script. We do not do and say the exact same thing every day. What is important is that the transition to resting happens in a calm and orderly manner. It is reassuring for someone with dementia to understand what we want him or her to do, to sense we have good intentions, and to be allowed to choose to take a rest. These factors are vital leading up to a rest, because drowsiness can feel overwhelming and strangely uncomfortable, like losing one's grip on reality.

This same process repeats several times a day, whenever a resident needs to rest. Most of the residents nap together, aligned in a row of single beds or reclining chairs next to each other in our resting room, which is normally bathed in light from the sunshine coming through the windows. It may seem strange to allow residents to rest side by side, but over time we have discovered that it makes them feel safe. I think they sense each other sleeping, with the sound of calm breathing and snoring. I also think it reflects a kind of social norm: "Everyone here is sleeping, so I had better sleep, too." Moreover, they sense that the staff are present and are looking after them in case anything arises. They can hear us working in the kitchen and walking around the living room.

During these naps, the residents sleep in the sunlight, with only a thin white curtain shading them from the sun. The light has a therapeutic effect while they are sleeping, stimulating their inner light, their optimism, and their relation to daylight.

They understand that this is not a nighttime sleep; it is only a nap. We do everything we can to make the residents feel grounded.

The residents seldom skip this rest in the middle of the day. For the most part, everyone sleeps 1–2 hours after lunch. More than half of the residents rest collectively, and the others get some peace and quiet in their own room. However, we tuck all of the residents in for a nap in the same manner, regardless of where they sleep.

Sleep patterns vary from resident to resident, and the need for rest depends on how each person has been affected by dementia and how much and what type of stimulation he or she can handle. The need for sleep can be a sign of how far the person's dementia has progressed. Some residents need to rest before lunch, right after, and later in the afternoon. Others only need the nap around noon.

A house with residents who have a healthy circadian rhythm is a house without major disruptions, without serious behavioral issues, and with a surplus of energy in both individual residents and the group as a whole. It is a home with a normal, cozy atmosphere.

Utilizing the circadian rhythm is not always as straightforward as it sounds. First of all, it can be difficult for some residents to fall into a good rhythm. These are often the residents who wake up at night. As much as possible, we keep them awake throughout the day, busily engaged with different activities. We try to limit the number of lighter, shorter "naps" that occur when residents sit and doze off; instead, they need to have real, long naps, often making do with one nap after lunch. When we want to adjust a sleep pattern so the resident sleeps through the night, we use physical activity, which keeps the resident awake and alert throughout the day. In addition to activity, we use a strategy of gradually keeping the person awake just a little longer each day, and after a couple of days or weeks he or she most often ends up sleeping through the night.

We have to be steadfast with regard to a resident's sleep. For instance, if a person is overtired and anxious as a result

Life at Our Home

Everyone has his or her own daily bedtime rituals. These rituals can seem unusual to those of us who care for people with dementia, but it is nevertheless important to discover them and accommodate them as much as possible. One of our residents had a difficult time napping in the middle of the day. But his dementia was so severe he needed the daytime rest. When he didn't nap, he would become easily stressed and aggressive. We could not understand his verbal communication, so we had to put on our detective hats and figure out what rituals he was trying to tell us he needed. We were able to convince him to lie down on the sofa, and we gave him a nice pillow and wrapped him in a soft wool blanket. We spoke softly to him and tried to relax him, but 2 minutes later he jumped to his feet again. He got more and more frustrated, pointing at things, trying to explain with words that made no sense. After a couple of days of trying one thing after another, one of our staff members discovered that, although he wanted us to remove his shoes while napping, he wanted to keep them next to his feet under the blanket. We wondered if he was afraid someone would take them and put them someplace where he would not be able to find them. In any case, once we began placing his shoes next to his feet, he no longer had any problems napping in the middle of the day. Finally sensing we understood him, he felt he could rest safely.

of that, we may have to sit on the edge of the bed until he or she drifts off. Everyone has different strategies for helping the residents fall asleep; these may include creating a peaceful atmosphere or something more stimulating, such as applying gentle pressure on the "third eye," the acupressure point between the eyebrows or on the forehead, to calm their racing thoughts. The care partner might also whisper words such as, "It's time to rest, and there's all the time in the world. I'll come back and check on you, and I'll be nearby the whole time." There are many ways to approach the situation, based on the individual staff member's own best judgment and the needs of the resident. It is just another example of how we are always working at full throttle, slowly.

The Norm: Good Morning?

At many care homes, there is no such thing as a circadian rhythm. The most obvious sign of this is that the residents do not have morning routines. Mornings are often reserved for the staff to come to work and gradually get started on the day's tasks. The residents who wake up easily get out of bed by themselves and are more or less ready at the normal breakfast time, somewhere between 8:00 and 10:00 a.m. The shared living areas are empty and desolate during the first hours of daylight.

Meanwhile, the more disabled and less engaged residents may be left to lie in bed much longer. When they finally get out of bed, their first activity is a kind of combined breakfast and lunch. They have no sense of time or rhythm to their day, which must be disheartening when you consider how many of them are from a generation that valued getting an early start. Instead, a plastic tray is hurriedly dropped off at each room, along with a cup of coffee from the machine.

What is lacking is a simple morning ritual, with the residents starting the day sitting together, taking in the dawning day. In many care homes, the residents' days are defined by randomness. When you peer into the care home's shared living room in the late morning, everything you observe is completely arbitrary. You might see a man half-sleeping in a corner, another stumbling in the hallway wearing slippers, a third with his pants half down, and a fourth at the dining table with a dry cheese sandwich. The staff member is next door, preoccupied with things she apparently could not leave to someone else. Static crackles from the radio by the windowsill. The lights are beaming with as many watts as possible. And this is what it looks like, day in and day out. The residents might have switched places, but you can count on them wearing the same clothes as the last time you were there.

After everyone is up, the day's potpourri of activities unfolds. In a distant corner, a loud staff member tries to facilitate an activity. The more restless residents are busy moving furniture. I wonder what the living room will look like when the evening team arrives. Here and there, more residents sit down and doze off in the chairs, even though it actually makes a difference, for both their body and their mind, whether they sleep lying down or sitting up.

You seldom see any scheduled resting times at care homes, nor any regular, daily program of activities. On the contrary, as evening rolls around, the residents merely look on as the staff quickly distribute their dinner. Then, they wait, as if on an assembly line, to be put to bed. This may occur according to their room number more often than their sleep requirements. The randomness enterprise just keeps ticking. Similar to the lack of cohesion in the morning, there are no evening rituals, either—not even something as obvious as eating together or watching television as a group. Nothing is planned to round off the day or help the residents to unwind. Care home staff are encouraged to concern themselves more with efficiency of movement: "If you're going down that way to put Karen in bed, could you also take care of Bent next door?" Staff members roll wheelchairs around from the living room down to the residents' rooms, hoist the resident up and down, turn off the light, and hurry out the door. Whether Karen or Bent actually needed to go to bed at this hour is not important.

What are the residents thinking, alone in the dark in their hospital beds? Can they process the day's experiences? Are they having happy thoughts? Who knows? No one has spent enough time with them to find out.

When I say that sleep can be important for treating dementia, staff often respond by claiming, "We've got a set routine." But when we actually discuss what that looks like, I learn more about how long the staff are on duty than about the needs of the residents. Most places completely disregard the importance of sleep for residents. A daily rhythm can develop only when the staff start keeping track of what is happening now. A daily rhythm prevents a random approach to the resident's life. A program suited to the needs of the residents is one that follows/is in accordance with their sleep cycles, and that highlights shared rituals in between periods of rest.

Objection:
"We let them sleep as long as they want."

We are doing a disservice to our residents if we let them sleep all morning. We should not assume people with dementia do not have the same need as we do—to have something to get up for. It is not good for our residents to lie in bed until noon. They should preferably be up before 9 a.m., because they need to sense that it is early in the morning, and to understand it as the start of a whole new day. Our schedule is always full, and the residents need to get a calm, orderly, and peaceful start.

> *We should not assume people with dementia do not have the same need as we do—to have something to get up for.*

If the residents get up late in the day and are then rolled into the shared living room for a sloppy mixture of breakfast and lunch, they start drifting indifferently, which makes life hard for someone who has dementia. In practical terms, if the person is not up and about before late morning, there is not much time left for participating in activities. In the next chapter, I describe our basic routine at Dagmarsminde.

One of the advantages of not letting residents sleep late is that you have residents who actually want to engage in daily activities and in all the new things happening around them. It helps them to progress—to the benefit of the staff as well. Energetic and participating residents both require the staff to think creatively and challenge them professionally, which makes their work both more fun and inspiring. It is nice to sit congenially with your colleagues over coffee while things are quiet down the hall, but I firmly believe most employees would prefer working with residents who demand something from them professionally. Our residents say the most fantastic, unexpected things and they make us feel lucky to be a part of this wonderful and incredible little world. Emphasizing the importance of sleep for the residents and mapping out and working with their individual circadian rhythms is of benefit not only to the residents themselves, but also to the staff, who will be more engaged and inspired by them.

Summary

At Dagmarsminde, we help our residents find and maintain a steady circadian rhythm in their lives. This effort is a combination of paying attention to the patterns of each individual person and encouraging the residents to move through the day in rhythm with each other. Living in a rhythm allows us to notice changes in a person's condition more readily, or notice new needs or problems quickly. Our residents enjoy the day's activities because they have more energy and feel more engaged and interested in life, which makes it much easier for us to create a positive, trusting relationship with them.

———•◆•———

Questions for Reflection

1. To what extent does your workplace encourage a regular, daily rhythm with a balance of sleep time and activities, as described in this chapter?

2. How do you weigh the sleep needs of an individual person in your care with the procedures and constraints imposed by the organization?

3. What, if anything, would have to change in your organization in order to ensure that your residents are getting the rest they need for optimal alertness and engagement throughout the day?

10

◆◇◆

The Routine

Together from Morning till Night

WE HAVE TO BE AHEAD of the game all of the time in order to create a daily flow, make the residents feel comfortable, and set the staff free. We do this by having a set routine—ideally, an ambitious one, with lots of goals. At Dagmarsminde, we plan every hour of the day, down to the smallest detail, so everyone knows what is going to happen and what each of us needs to contribute. In this way, we can enable the activities as they come. Whether you use this chapter as a template or merely as inspiration, the main point is the importance of establishing a daily routine, because that is the foundation for building a life of ease and comfort for your residents.

Daily Routine

Early Morning

Getting an early start is crucial. Our days begin as the overnight team meets between 7:00 and 8:00 a.m. to hand over care to the morning team. The night team provides an overview of the preceding night: how the residents slept, whether anyone was restless, who got up, and so on. Having this overview helps us know what to expect during the day. We never linger at the morning meeting; we get to work straightaway.

Before the handover meeting, the night team has usually already helped four of our residents out of bed. This allows enough time for each individual resident's morning care routine, and sufficient time is vital for our residents. We cannot hurry them out of bed or into the shower. We let them go at their own pace, choose their own clothes, and hold their own showerhead or washcloth. We allow the whole process to take the time it needs—even the way they wake up. We might sit by a person's bedside for a while, or offer a glass of fresh juice. From the moment he or she wakes up, the resident needs to sense—even in the occasional moment of confusion—that the person sitting with them only has good intentions. A staff member stays in the shared living room with those residents who are already up and are either contentedly waiting at the breakfast table or lying down in the rest area.

By about 8:30 a.m., all residents have been helped out of bed. There is time for a shower if the resident feels like it; washing is not reserved for certain days of the week just because it fits the schedule. Everyone is dressed and helped to the shared living space, where a well-spread breakfast table is waiting for them with freshly baked bread, coffee, and tea. We always sit together when we eat.

Around 9:00 a.m., we have all finished eating, and staff members begin to prepare the group for a walk outside. By 9:30 a.m., we have all been—or still are—in the garden. We usually walk in small groups, making sure that all the residents get outside, at least for a little while. We take a walk to look at the animals and discuss what we see. Some of the residents sit down on a bench in the sun; others want to go right back inside again, especially if it is windy outside. Nevertheless, everyone needs to get outside for some fresh air, even just for a quick round. Residents with severe dementia seldom enjoy being outside for very long. In general, they only stay outside long enough to feel a breeze and the sun on their face, or a couple of drops on their skin if it is drizzling.

During the cold months, our garden walks are usually limited to 15–20 minutes. In the spring, summer, or warm autumn days, we sometimes stay out much longer, doing our daily reading or our exercises outside. But for most of the year, we come inside again and sit on the sofas in the shared living room for our reading after our walk. Moving to a different setting helps define the new activity, making it easier for the residents to focus on what happens next. A staff member sits in the middle of the sofas and reads to the residents. At various points, she might ask them questions about what she is reading or start a discussion. Generally, this reading period lasts from 9:30 to 10:30 a.m.

Those residents who cannot keep still for so long may wander back and forth to the sofas or go lie down in the resting area. But most find the reading period pleasurable, and they are quietly attentive while the staff member reads. It is calm and peaceful; we have a rule during this hour that staff should not make any noise in the kitchen or talk in the background. The conditions need to be optimal for the residents to be carried away into whatever world the reader is describing. It might be an extract of travel writing, a biography, or an adventure story. Ensuring a quiet environment is key. It enables the residents to really listen and absorb the material, letting the words linger and picturing the images, and letting their minds wander to another, perhaps unknown, time. The reading, if done without disturbances in the background, has a powerful effect on the residents. A staff member who is present but is not reading makes sure everything remains calm, by talking quietly to residents who are distracting others, or helping them out for a walk outside. This background attention allows the reader to focus on engaging the listening residents.

Life at Our Home

How do we know if the residents are listening at reading time? It's simple. The first 15 minutes usually include some subtle stirring, a bit of chitchat, someone reaching out for a glass of water, or residents scanning the room. That's okay at the start, but if the disturbances continue or increase, then the material might be too difficult to grasp or may just not be that entertaining. We know our own residents, and we know which one can let us know if the material is working or not. We have one resident who, in the middle of the reading, will ask what we are doing afterward if she isn't being sufficiently entertained. Conversely, if she is actively engaged in the book and the reader pauses too long between paragraphs, she will impatiently say, "Why are you stopping?" In this way, she serves as a kind of spokesperson for the group; we use her lack of filter to our advantage and can tell whether our listeners are following us or we have lost their attention.

Late Morning

Once the residents have eaten breakfast, gone outside, and had coffee, tea, or a glass of water or juice during the reading, they usually need to go to the bathroom. We spend some time after the reading helping everyone to the toilet before our exercises, which start at 10:30 a.m. and last about an hour. We do our aerobic exercises in our shared living space. As described in Chapter 6, we lead the residents in different kinds of exercises: muscle strengthening, cardiovascular training, and coordination and memory exercises. We also hold question-and-answer sessions, in which we ask the residents who they are and what kind of work they did, where they come from, and so on, but using the present tense throughout, as if they are still working (otherwise, many of them can get confused). We might also come up with a name game, so the residents practice saying each other's names and our names. Besides a memory practice, this is also a way of reiterating that the people they see around them right now are the same people they see every day. By the way, we never use name tags; we feel that those are too institutional. Instead, we always say our name before we walk into a resident's room: "Hi, it's me, Dorte. I'm coming in . . ."

Midday

Our shared lunchtime is at 11:30 a.m. Shortly before then, we end our exercises with a dance or two. It is almost a ritual for our residents to sanitize their hands with a dab of antibacterial lotion before lunch. When we are done eating, at around 12:30 p.m., most of the residents feel like resting. We help them over to our resting room, a sunroom, for their noontime nap. Some of them will want to sleep in their own room, but most of them are in the resting room or on one of the three sofas in our shared living room.

On the whole, the residents are very willing to lie down to nap, and, after another bathroom visit, they quickly fall asleep. Then the home is generally quiet until about 2:30 p.m. During this time, the staff tidy the kitchen, set the table for coffee, fold napkins, and put the cake in the oven that the overnight team has prepared in advance. This napping period also allows time for the staff to note down the day's observations so far. Once a week, we use this time for a longer meeting, which we call our board meeting, to discuss the condition of all of the residents.

Afternoon

At around 2:30 p.m., we wake up the residents. Some of them may already be up and about. We welcome them back to the community with the delightful smell of cake wafting through the shared rooms. After a trip to the bathroom, the residents gather at the main table, where we have cake and tea or coffee with them. Around this time, any visiting relatives will join us around the table.

After several larger group gatherings throughout the day, residents need a break in the schedule. Breaks are key to calmly and naturally drawing the resident's attention back into other shared activities. This is why, at about 3:30, we invite our residents to go outside again for a little while to allow them to walk around together or on their own. Then, at about 4:00 p.m., we bring them inside for another session in the sofa area that includes either reading, singing, or conversation. The reason for this session, between 4:00 and 5:30 p.m., is that this is the time of day people with dementia often become restless.

During this time we also prepare their dinner and set the table. There are only two staff members working during these hours of the day. So, while one of them is setting a beautiful dinner table, the other is with the residents. When the session is done, the residents are escorted to the bathroom. Around then, a third staff member joins us, and is on duty for the next 4 hours.

Evening

At about 5:30, we turn on some music and invite the residents to dinner, which begins around 5:45 p.m. We serve a warm dinner and sit around the table for about 45 minutes. A staff member arranges the food nicely on the plates and serves them, while the two others ensure a calm and cozy atmosphere around the table.

By 6:30 p.m., the residents are enjoying the evening in front of the television, where we offer them some coffee, tea, and a little dessert. We watch the news. Afterward, they might see a film. The evening staff have discovered that the residents are intrigued by programs such as opera, ballet, and classical music or choir concerts. Our television is hooked up to a couple of high-quality speakers, which enhances the experience of these more artistic, cultural shows. Yet we never sit for too long because most of the residents are clearly worn out by this time.

Around 8:00 p.m., many of the residents are so tired they want to go to sleep. For the most part, they have been awake since the early morning and are definitely ready for bed. We help them into bed one by one, following each person's own pace as much as possible.

One staff member always stays behind with the residents remaining in the living room. This is one of our policies, which must be followed at all times throughout the day; problems can arise in the blink of an eye if someone is not watching over people with dementia. An unsteady resident might suddenly decide to get up, or another resident might become frustrated and angry.

Nighttime

Before bedtime, one of the staff members checks each room, making sure it is ready, removing bedcovers, cracking open the window, and placing a hot-water bottle in the bed so that it is warm when the resident lies down. The residents like this last item and might keep the bottle next to them all night. Every resident has his or her own nightly rituals, which help put their minds at ease. One resident may need us to sit with her on the edge of her bed and talk; another may need some leg massage.

Almost everyone is in bed by 10:00 p.m. The evening staff take this time to tidy the house, complete the daily journals, and hang up the rest of the laundry. They typically finish between 11:00 and 11:30 p.m., when the overnight team arrives. A slight overlap is scheduled between all of the shifts, and when staff arrive for any shift, they start by reading what happened that day, evening, or night.

Overnight

The night staff have their own set schedule and tasks to perform. They prepare the house for the next morning. They set the table, bake rolls, cut fruit for breakfast, iron smocks, put fresh candles in the candelabra, and so on. Three times per night, they check on the sleeping residents. This inspection does not disrupt the residents; rather, it adds to their sense of security. If a resident wakes up, the staff member takes the time to comfort him or her. If those efforts are not effective, the staff member brings the person to the living room and invites him or her to lie down in the resting area. Here, the person usually falls asleep again, sensing the night staff are nearby. Sometimes, though, it is enough for the staff to fetch the cat and let it sleep on the resident's bed.

All of our rooms have a sensor so that we can hear if a resident tries to get up and can quickly go help him or her relax again. By using a sensor in this way, we do not have to worry about residents wandering around, in danger of falling or feeling lost, confused, or anxious. This is one technological development that I actually find helpful. It is an assistive device, but it should never become a replacement for real inspections. The overnight staff still enter every room to determine if everything is okay. They have to sense whether the temperature is alright and whether the resident is breathing calmly and resting in a correct position. As mentioned previously, around 6:00 a.m., the overnight employees start helping some of our early risers out of bed.

Excursions

Sometimes I am asked whether we go on excursions with the residents. We do not do this very often. We might take a drive to the beach or down to the local harbor, but our residents cannot handle a trip to Copenhagen's central entertainment park, Tivoli, for instance. There is too much stimulation, and long trips do not allow for the necessary periods of rest. Besides this, the residents never request excursions. In our experience, they are most comfortable staying and following a known routine at our little oasis.

The Norm:
"Bingo's been cancelled."

Many care homes have some sort of weekly activities, listed in the latest resident newsletter. For instance, a home might schedule Bingo on Tuesday, a prayer service on Wednesday, men's billiards on Friday. Certain days are reserved for certain scheduled activities. What the residents spend their time doing during the unscheduled hours, however, is a mystery. The leaders of these homes prefer to deal with activities on a day-to-day basis. Instead of having a set schedule, perhaps they have jotted down some fluffy-sounding slogan about activities being part of their core values; if the slogan is not hanging in a frame at the entrance, it is probably still on a shelf in someone's office. Maybe you have seen these types of slogans: "Rose Garden care home is an active and stimulating care home."

The problem is that many homes do not live up to these values. The good intentions are not actually carried out as part of a daily schedule. We cannot just make a pledge to offer activities, tasks, and meeting times, and then stand by and watch as it unravels. Often, the sensory garden and the care home's other stimulating features sit waiting for someone to actually use them. A fixed schedule is imperative to being able to follow through with your promises.

For example, when a care home states, "On Tuesday we have Bingo," it is often more a symbolic gesture, which is typical of institutional thinking. They are saying, "Look, we're doing something for the residents." But in reality, these kinds of random amusements only accentuate the care home's lack of planning for the *rest* of the day. It is a far cry from a daily schedule. When the resident newsletter states, "Once a month we enjoy a nice brunch together," we have good reason to be skeptical. As it turns out, the culinary event offers the same indistinct scrambled eggs served at any other day's mix of breakfast/lunch/dinner, at whatever hour the resident is helped out of bed. The "brunch" in this case is just another cover for the care home's lack of structure.

In the many hours and days when nothing in particular is scheduled, both the staff and the residents are directionless. When you consider how planning and organization are the backbone of every thriving business and every good school as well as every successful journey, why would we not take the time to organize the days and hours of people with dementia living in a care home?

Besides the lack of planned activities, many care homes are afflicted with what I call "staff cancellation readiness." For these homes, it takes very little disruption for them to cancel their hyped-up activities. Perhaps the activity leader is sick, or not enough residents checked their names on the list on the notice board. "We'll play Bingo some other time," a staff member sighs with relief. But did anyone step forward to encourage residents to sign up or offer to help them move out of their rooms and over to where Bingo is played?

Someone with dementia is no longer able to process such thoughts and actions as, "I'd like to play Bingo on Tuesday, so I had better sign up now. Let me find a pen." That person needs our assistance. That is what it means to be dependent. As staff, we can either choose to oblige that dependence or exploit it. Only the staff can encourage and help residents to participate in scheduled plans. Yet no one objects to arbitrary cancellations because everyone assumes these elders are better off without too many events and should have the right to sleep late in the name of self-determination. This lackadaisical attitude reflects the low expectations we often have for the elders in our care—at least in Denmark, which is ironically one of the world's wealthiest welfare countries due to residents like ours having contributed for half a century.

The message here is simple: Do not just randomly offer a bunch of isolated activities. Have a set plan. A day needs to be a series of connected, repeating activities, so that the day itself becomes a familiar rhythmic feature in the residents' lives.

Benefits of a Consistent Schedule

It is actually much better for everyone if things unfold steadily within a planned schedule. Most people who do not have dementia have a daily routine. We get up, drive the kids to school and ourselves to work, go home, make dinner, watch television, and so on. There is a natural rhythm to most of our lives, which is how it should also be for care home residents, as well as the staff and the families of the residents.

> *Because of the daily schedule, we have time for the*
> *individual resident in between the shared activities.*

For example, it is important to know that when you visit your aging relative at 10:00 a.m. today, he or she is probably strolling around the garden with the other residents. Or maybe you know that it is better to wait until after 10:00 a.m. because the person is usually resting between 9:00 and 10:00. A daughter of one of our residents described that what our schedule means to her is that her mother is doing something enriching at all times. Every time she drives up our driveway, she thinks, "I can't wait to see what my mom is up to."

Objection:
"Isn't that a bit rigid?"

Some people wrinkle their noses at the idea of having a set schedule at their care home. "How can we accommodate for individual needs with that kind of schedule?" I always remind them that managing a care home will never be a military operation, but that as soon as they incorporate a daily schedule, the value of doing so will become self-evident. Because of the daily schedule, we have time for the individual resident in between the shared activities. The detailed planning creates not only time but also surplus energy to tend to the needs of the individuals in our care.

Most of the residents enjoy being part of a community. Having one staff member assigned to lead an activity of a larger group, such as exercises or reading out loud, gives another staff member time to attend to a resident with special needs on that day. In this way, the schedule enables flexibility. Without a schedule, we would have residents moving in all directions, with all sorts of issues arising at the same time. It is virtually impossible to attend to so many needs at once. This kind of chaos can lead to irritation and stress, as well as an increased risk of unnecessary medicating. By comparison, perhaps a daily schedule is not so rigid after all.

A daily schedule also supports the residents' circadian rhythm. Setting a daily schedule for the residents means they naturally get tired in the evening and sleep longer and more deeply throughout the night. They are more energetic, healthier, and easier to work with the next morning. Also, we almost never have residents who take a long time to get out of bed. In general, they have all had a good night's sleep and are ready to seize the day. A set schedule makes it easier to get them up.

Summary

Some might contend that, considering the age and dementia of the residents, it is meaningless to enforce these kinds of strict schedules. But we believe these people still have a life and a future, and that they deserve to get the most out of it just like the rest of us. Every aspect of the care work we perform, including setting and adhering to a schedule, reflects that belief.

———— •◆• ————

Questions for Reflection

1. Consider the daily or weekly schedule at your organization. Is it closer to the approach used at Dagmarsminde or is it closer to how the author describes "the norm"? List examples of each.

2. Do you agree with the author's argument that having a set schedule could actually allow for more flexibility? Explain why or why not.

3. Are there ideas presented in this chapter that you would like to see implemented in part or in whole at your care home? List the steps needed for that to happen.

11

Sanatorium Practices

WHEN WE THINK OF A sanatorium, we imagine people from a hundred years ago, rehabilitating in beautiful surroundings. Before the discovery of antibiotics, the best-known treatment for tuberculosis—although not a cure—consisted of fresh air, sunlight, and different types of exercise. Sanatoria were usually located near forests and mountains, with the understanding that peace and quiet in the presence of nature were essential for successful treatment. And, indeed, the quality of the patients' lives improved. Ever since I first saw old photographs of patients lying in the sun under giant arches or resting in a courtyard garden, I have been inspired by this approach, which has existed for centuries all over the world. It makes sense to bring back these ideas and merge them with our treatment for those who have dementia, for whom there is no medical cure. Given that we do not want medicine to be the primary form of treatment anyway, what better place to introduce this mindset than our care home?

Pampering to Heal

The sanatorium approach can go hand in hand with a professional nursing perspective. This approach involves using fresh air and the natural world in your care work—having residents bathe in sunlight. Our job is to offer the residents healing and alleviate their symptoms; therefore, in addition to the presence of nature, we spice up the older sanatorium ideas with a little modern pampering to make the residents feel special. Pampering is a big part of what we do.

At Dagmarsminde, we created a little spa area to integrate the ideas of the past into our care. Our spa area is designed to fit a warm-water therapy pool (4 × 6 meters), lounge chairs, a massage table, lots of green plants, bamboo lamps with a soft light, and a sound system for playing meditative music and nature sounds. We bring in residents one at a time to boost their well-being and pamper them. This is the room where the residents can sense, "It's all about me now."

I often get questions about how we use it, how it benefits the residents—and even more so, how we make time for this "addition" to standard care. It is important to remember that our spa services are not just for the residents' well-being; they also enhance cleanliness and help prevent infections.

Warm-Water Therapy Pool

Some of our residents are able to enter our therapy pool using the steps. For others, we use a lift to lower the residents down into the 96°F water. This requires two staff members: One is positioned in the water, ready to receive the resident, while the other controls the lift, explaining the process to the resident as it is underway. It is essential to review this with the resident many times and in different ways; some of them can get a little scared as we lower them into the water. In general, though, they quickly calm down and relax once they are in the water. Sometimes they even fall asleep in the water, still strapped to the sling, which can feel as snug as a hammock. The resident relaxes and feels weightless. We believe the feeling of weightlessness is significant for our residents; in this state, they feel that they are neither a burden nor that they are burdened.

Fifteen minutes in the water is our usual rule. Otherwise, the heat can get too intense for the person. The only challenge is when a resident does not want to get out. We might offer a glass of cold juice and help him or her get dressed. After this dip in the water, the person is often exhausted, and it is a good time for a nap.

Occasionally, we have two or three women in the pool together, and they may splash and play a bit. But if a resident cannot stand up in the water without help, then only that person and a staff member are permitted in the water at a given time.

The warm water in the pool can be enormously soothing. It feels good, is comforting, and relaxes the residents' ligaments and muscles. We have had particularly positive experiences with those residents who have Parkinson's disease and whose bodies are very stiff. A chronically clenched fist is suddenly able to release and open completely. Water works wonders on a body, and the gentle lapping sound of water has a calming effect on the mind.

The residents do not go into the pool every day. It is a special activity, which needs to fit with whatever else is going on. The staff member on duty needs at least half an hour at

Life at Our Home

We recently helped one of our residents, who is constantly restless and "in her own world," into our therapy pool. Her language is unintelligible, and her sense of space and short-term memory have been greatly affected by her condition. After entering the water, she just sat there for a little while. We made a conscious effort not to talk to her, letting the room be filled with the sound of a single cello playing on our loudspeakers. Then, seated on the step and talking nonstop in her own language, she began churning the water with her arms swimming. After a couple of minutes, she suddenly said very clearly, "Grandmother loves being by the water." Much later that same day, the staff noticed that she repeatedly referred to "Grandmother's" experience at the pool, saying things like "the water feels wonderful" and "Grandmother has been swimming."

her disposal. But with a little ingenuity, we manage, and the residents frequently take a dip in the pool. Some of them use the pool a couple of times a week, while others only use it once a month or even less often.

For some residents, their general condition vastly improves after a dip in the water. When their muscles are particularly tense, the relaxing effect lingers long into the day. The residents become more comfortable in their own skin when we use the warm-water treatment on a regular basis.

Many people ask me if using a pool is not all just a hassle. It does require extra energy to organize around its use and to ensure that it becomes a regular activity, but really it is not difficult. Another concern I hear is about loose stools in the water. Let me reassure you, we do not have any issues with loose stools when our residents are in the water. We make sure they have been to the bathroom before they go in the water, and if there is a risk of this problem, they use a swimsuit designed to avoid water contamination. Most important is that care partners want to work with the residents in the water. Being in the pool with a resident is a unique experience that strengthens the bond between the staff member and the resident.

Spa Services

Besides the therapy pool, we also use the spa area to give the residents massages, manicures, facials, and acupuncture treatments. The function of the manicure is primarily to maintain the residents' nails, but of course the women often love an occasional coat of red polish. We have to make sure the residents do not develop ingrown nails, which can get infected, and we have to avoid letting their nails grow so long they harbor dirt or bacteria. Massaging the muscles in the palm of their hand, which are often surprisingly tender, also works wonders. With similar benefits, we provide the residents foot therapy every sixth week, and the services of a hairdresser as needed. The sanatorium practices, as mentioned, also incorporate the use of nature, which will be discussed in more detail in Chapter 12.

When we have time to give a facial, it is not only for special treatment and pampering. Stimulating a person's skin
with moisture and massage can make them look radiant and
raise their self-esteem. The women, especially, feel "dainty"
afterward.

Central to all of these services is the residents' health.
When we have a basic understanding of the traditional sanatorium principles, then we take a word like *healing* seriously.

When I describe to others the way we work, I am
often asked if our approach would be manageable within
the framework of a "normal" nursing home run by a state,
church, or corporation. The answer is yes, as long as you
do not assume the treatment has to be the same for everyone. We do charge extra fees for some of our services that
are not covered under state requirements or insurance. The
residents' families understand that they have to pay for some
special treatments themselves. At Dagmarsminde, all residents have their nails cut and basic grooming taken care of
by the staff, but pampering facials, massage for the hands
and feet, cuticle treatment, and other aesthetic services, for
example, are financed by the residents themselves or by their
relatives. The rest of our sanatorium treatments, such as the
pool, massage, and footbaths are a just a regular part of our
everyday care. We believe that is what caring is all about.

The Norm:
"You're more than welcome to get a haircut . . ."

Some care homes say they offer haircuts, manicures, massages,
or warm-water treatments, but often it is up to the relatives to
not only pay for but facilitate these services. They are not considered the care home's responsibility, so they often do not happen. But organizing these types of services should never be left
to the relatives. They should not have to phone the barber or or
coordinate other appointments. Their job is to offer their love
and support for their loved one. They should be able to devote

all of their time and attention to relating to their family member, which can be complicated at times, considering that their loved one's personality may have changed. We must ensure that relatives have the time and space to be close to their loved ones.

Many relatives know that clean, well-kept hands are a rarity at nursing homes. Nails grow and become long, crooked, and dirty. Although it is trendy for staff to paint the residents' fingernails, the nails might not be properly cleaned or manicured first, so the polish goes on over layers of dirt, and the nails may be lumpy and ingrown. The focus is on the pretty polish, not basic hygiene. When the motivation for these kinds of initiatives is not founded in the sanatorium principles, then the care home might as well not offer them, because they do not benefit the residents' health. These services have to be based on principles of good health and need to be provided on a regular basis.

Objection:
"Residents will ask for more."

If the sanatorium ideas are taken seriously and spa treatments are a regular part of care, then what usually happens is that the residents start making demands. This is actually a healthy sign, because it means that the old feelings of defeat from the past have been washed away, and the person is rediscovering his or her own basic needs and desires. However, the general mindset among many in our care sector is that care home residents should not be making demands. The residents of care homes are considered to be heading toward the edge anyway, especially those who have dementia, who aren't considered to be able to benefit from these services. And besides, "they are old and have had their joys" is the attitude.

But the elderly, *like the rest of us*, enjoy feeling clean and comfortable. Older women still like maintaining their skin and hands, getting their hair cut and blow-dried, and plucking out those coarse hairs that sometimes grow on their faces. Yet it is not uncommon to see women at nursing homes with facial hair, greasy hair, waxen skin, and looking overall unkempt—or men with thick, ingrown nails and stubble on their faces.

Summary

What do you do when you are feeling tired, worn down, and need some pampering? Do you take a yoga class, get some coaching, or maybe even sign up for a weekend getaway at a spa? These are experiences many of us dream of after a stressful couple of weeks at work. Why should we not offer people with dementia the same opportunities for special treatment? They might even need it even more than we do. If caring is about showing empathy, then we have to shelve the idea of the same equal standard for everyone. Some people need more pampering than others—people with dementia, in particular.

————•◆•————

Questions for Reflection

1. What kinds of spa services are offered at your care home? Are they primarily aesthetic services or more health-focused?

2. Do you feel that your organization operates from an understanding of sanatorium principles, as described by the author? Why or why not?

3. Take an imaginary, or real, walk through the halls of your care home. Observe the faces, skin, and nails of the residents you see. How do they look, in general? What can you learn about the state of their overall health by observing them in this way?

12

---•◆•---

The Great Outdoors

Sensing at the Highest level

IN CHAPTER 8, I SHARED how we see people as part of a bigger picture. In this chapter, I outline how we actually put these ideas into practice and use the natural world as part of our care on a daily basis. Every day, I see what being outdoors does for our residents—and our staff. At Dagmarsminde, we are lucky to have both a garden right outside our door and an inspiring and diverse old forest close by.

To the Forest

We go to the forest as often as possible. Some months, we go several times a week, and less frequently at other times of the year. We prefer going when it is dry, sunny, and not too windy, but because that is usually too much to ask for in Denmark, we also go on gray, cloudy days. The only times we do not go are when it is stormy or pouring down rain, because that kind of weather can be stressful for the residents. They are easily overwhelmed by the forces of nature.

As we head off to the woods, anyone passing will see us either pushing the residents in wheelchairs or guiding them on foot down the gravelly path toward the forest. Once we are in the forest, we are surrounded by something bigger and stronger than ourselves, as well as something deeply harmonious. The forest can be sensitive, and at times, melancholic. All around us are trees of all different shapes and sizes. The trees offer us both shade and sunshine and a feeling of protection. The forest floor crunches softly under our feet, the ground is uneven, and the sounds fill our hearts with joy.

The forest is a mecca of sensory experience. The residents roam around the unfamiliar terrain. They have to be careful where they step, and it can be challenging for them. We open our eyes and venture deeper down the little paths or in between the towering beech trees. Sometimes, we pick a tree and decide to take a closer look. We walk up to it, touch it, and feel its bark without too much talking. We might ask the resident, "Which tree would you like to look at?" It is a rewarding intuitive exercise, in which we nurture the resident's connection to nature. We might even do the exercise with everyone on the little expedition as a group. We gather in a circle around the tree, talk about the tree, and feel a shared togetherness. We mean it when we say that the tree is "conscious" and a part of us.

Some might say we sound like a bunch of hippies. But the residents enjoy it. A couple of them might scoff a little as we start the session because they find it weird, but at the same time they like it. "Touch the bark here, what does it feel like?" we might ask, guiding their hands over to the tree. When we talk about the tree, they all join in. How old do you think this tree is? Why did that burl develop or how did it get those cuts? We can see the residents are touched by the experience. Their eyes light up, they sigh with relief, or their eyes well with tears. It stirs up all sorts of strong emotions.

When we talk about a tree, the conversation often leads to the residents and their own lives. The tree has a cut, but it healed. Once again, the focus is on increasing our awareness and consciousness. It is a holistic experience. We are here together in nature. We gather branches, bark, and flowers. We pick them up and examine them. The residents join in by themselves.

Sometimes we sit down beside the forest lake. We ask the residents to be silent for a few minutes so that everyone can listen to the sounds of the forest, smell it, and let themselves be enveloped by their sensory perceptions and the feeling of being a part of nature. Something special happens when we sit there together in the silence of a giant forest.

If you have worked with people who have dementia, you know how challenging it can be to get a group of them to be quiet and sit still. But in the forest, everything is easier. We might put an arm around a slightly restless resident and say gently, "Shh . . . try to be quiet for a moment. Try to listen to the forest." We show how to be quiet by whispering, or maybe we close our eyes in front of the resident. Suddenly, we are sitting in a close circle in a meditative state. We might sit there anywhere from 5 minutes to half an hour.

All sorts of devices have been invented for those who are frail or elderly, but there is nothing like a walk in the woods. Nature stimulates the residents while also putting their minds at ease in a whole new way. Each person in their own manner engages with the forest and is entirely absorbed by it. We always see development in the residents after a trip to the forest. They might start walking or speaking more clearly and coherently. Maybe the muscles in their face relax or there is an excited, youthful energy to them, as though they are somehow inebriated. In Japan, the practice of allowing trees to have an effect on the body and soul is called *forest bathing*.

Yet another important factor is that being in the forest is normalizing. In the forest, we are who we are. No one is categorized as a "care home resident." In the forest, we can all be ourselves. Perhaps that is also why the residents are able to open up and show their emotions. Back home at Dagmarsminde, they may acknowledge they are residents at a care home—but in the forest, their self-image is undefined. It is a completely different mindset, one might say, which allows them to see themselves as normal people. Human beings are natural beings, and experiencing the natural world is a fundamental human need. If your care home is not close to a forest, I encourage you to plan a trip to one, at least once in a while, to include these kinds of powerful experiences in your care program.

A Garden of Flora and Fauna

The garden is another essential feature of our care home. Gardens inspire people. We have spent years shaping our garden at Dagmarsminde, with flowers, bushes, and trees of different sizes.

We use the garden for short daily outings. It is somewhere to go, something to do. The garden provides a way to enjoy our natural surroundings and be inspired by beauty. It is also a place with purpose. Our garden is fenced in, so the residents are free to wander on their own. They go into and out of the garden every day, several times a day. In fact, there are very few days in the year when they do not go out there; only the snow or pouring rain can keep them inside.

An important part of our care treatment is giving the residents a sense of wholeness, stability, and strength. That is why we have placed different rocks in the garden for the residents to touch, lean against, sit on, or look at. In some ways, the garden is a kind of life force, imbuing a sense of connection.

> *We do everything in our power to arouse the resident's underlying, instinctual will to live.*

We are constantly developing our garden, with any funds available. Our mission is to create a space with continuous movement, a passageway that transitions into different experiences. The residents can pass in and out of the stone gates where we have made a pathway with smooth, rounded stones from Danish beaches. They can even go barefoot, stimulating important nerve pathways on the bottoms of their feet, as well as "grounding" them in a way people with dementia need. Our path, which also heightens their awareness, leads them into smaller areas where they can be alone or find focus in shared meditation.

While being led down a pathway, residents move their bodies more naturally than they would, for example, on an exercise machine. If they need to rest, they can sit down on one of the big, flat stones that have been placed to give them a view across fields stretching as far as the eye can see. Our little meditative area, with wide open spaces all around and Dagmarsminde right behind, gives them peace of mind. To balance out the fixed position and hardness of the stones with something delicate and mobile, we have planted different trees that bear fruit or flowers and that offer the shade of their leaves. Our hedges are left untrimmed. We have added colorful flowers that support biodiversity by attracting bees, butterflies, and insects. The soft world of flowers fills the air with scents and colors, awakening their optimism.

In the middle of the garden is our all-important firepit. We often gather around the fire, devoting our attention to the flames and embers. The fire in the middle of our circle offers us a rare experience of calm and reflection. The residents can sit and stare at the flames for a long time. As you might have guessed by now, we do everything in our power to arouse the resident's underlying, instinctual will to live.

We have chosen to include animals in our garden as well as inside our home because they have so much to offer our residents. We have goats, which are hand-fed by the residents and are also fun to watch and play with. When children or grandchildren come for a visit, they can share in the joy of the animals with their grandparents or great-grandparents.

The residents also help feed the chickens, and every day we collect the eggs in the chicken coop. The chickens are part of our little ecosystem; they eat our scraps and, in exchange, we use their eggs for our afternoon cakes or, occasionally, scrambled eggs for breakfast.

Life at Our Home

One summer, as I was crossing our garden at dusk with the flowers in bloom and the air still warm, I spotted three of our residents together without a staff member. They were standing by the chicken coop, clearly amused by the social interactions of the chickens. All 16 chickens crowded against the fence, competing for a spot near the residents and practically clucking in sync. I stayed back but picked up some of the residents' conversation. It struck me how completely normal their demeanor appeared; no one would ever have guessed they all had severe dementia. They stood with their backs straight, chatting as if they were attending a garden party. They shared polite remarks about keeping chickens and congratulated each other on having the foresight to buy them for the garden.

We also have rabbits—at the moment, six of them—and they are cute as they jump around in a long cage in the garden. Once in a while we bring them inside, for example when we read out loud to the residents, because they instill a sense of calm and focus. When a resident has a rabbit sitting on his or her lap, it is easier to stay seated and listen to the reading.

Often, our copper-colored Burmese cat Herman will lie on top of the residents when they are resting. Our lively red golden retriever Trolle might be seen stretched out on the floor near the entrance, waiting eagerly for someone to come scratch his belly. We sometimes enlist him for an enthusiastic morning call with a resident who is difficult to get up, or for comfort if a resident is sad. He also joins us for our walks in the garden. Both the cat and the dog motivate the residents to bend or squat down.

The features of a garden need to both strengthen the residents and bring them closer to nature. That is one of the reasons we do not aim for a highly groomed—or what I would call an "uptight"—garden, one you cannot engage with other than to admire from a distance. Much of the landscaping I have seen at nursing homes consists of little green areas with rows of plants like the ones you see in front of shopping centers. We are not invited to engage with them, and they are therefore uninteresting.

It is helpful to think about how a garden can stimulate people in order to be more intentional about the landscaping of a care home. A garden is important because it is the residents' only regular contact with the outside world and is a way for them to follow the seasonal changes. They have to be able to touch the grass, flowers, bushes, and trees. Just see what happens when you let the residents walk on the grass with their bare feet.

The Norm:
The "Stress Garden"

Many nursing homes advertise their "sensory gardens." Originally, a sensory garden was a place filled with herbs, scents of flowers in many different colors, and cozy spaces with tables and benches where you could soak up all the sights, sounds, and delights of the garden. Throughout history, hospitals have had these types of gardens on their grounds because sitting in the sun and experiencing the many things a garden has to offer can help rejuvenate people who are ill.

Unfortunately, the term sensory garden no longer seems to mean the same thing it did historically. Once the concept went mainstream, retailers took over, along with a wide range of merchandise. Once again, the care sector was swept off its feet by all the advances in technology, and these days gardens are filled with contraptions where the residents can push a button and hear music or nature sounds. I have even seen "dementia-friendly" plastic animals; residents can get up close and pet the "cows." It is simply deceptive.

Nursing homes will purchase expensive architect-designed "sensory furniture," such as outdoor sofa hammocks and swings. These are as hard for me to fathom as they are hard for the residents to get out of. The motto seems to be: "'Special' people need 'special' things." A sensory garden ends up becoming so *special*, the only thing the resident senses is how different he or she is from the rest of us. Many of these gardens are also outfitted like a gym, like those calisthenics parks for adults in big cities. Many of these so-called gardens are not really gardens at all. Regardless of whether they have been carefully designed or not, the gardens in most nursing homes are usually empty of people.

A family member of one of our residents told us about her experience with a different nursing home's attempt at a sensory garden.

In the spring of 2018, the nursing home celebrated the opening of their new sensory garden with the residents, the staff, and the relatives. There were flowers and bushes in raised beds, stone sculptures of little animals, and water gushing from the fountain in the middle of the garden. There was also champagne, cake, and a toast to everyone there. For seating, the garden had one specially designed outdoor sofa and an old bench that was there from before. All of the funds had gone into designing the garden, so there was no money left for new tables and extra benches where people could sit and enjoy the flowers. Unfortunately, too, it was not easily accessible to the residents, who had to take a long detour to get to it.

The summer was relatively dry that year, so many of the plants quickly withered. The relatives assumed the plants had not been watered because of the nationwide water-saving campaign that was going on back then. But the following spring, when they were looking forward to stepping out into the garden and seeing it replanted with spring flowers, the relatives found that nothing had happened. There were no signs of new plants, and weeds and briars gradually took over. The fountain looked equally forlorn.

Summer arrived, and the garden kept getting wilder and wilder, and no one ever visited it. One resident who lived on the second floor started calling it the "stress garden." It made him anxious because he once had had a beautiful garden that he constantly tended. When the relatives asked the administration about it, the reply was always: "We're trying to find out if it's the county or the housing association's responsibility." That was the reason the garden transformed into an unbridled mess, and no one wanted to use it.

It was only after local media were contacted that things started moving. Workers from the county, who it turns out were responsible for the garden, started redesigning it, almost from scratch. It took most of the summer to lay out the new sensory garden. The resident sat in his apartment, watching the gardeners working below, and said, "I wonder if I'll ever see it blossom." He never did. He died the following spring and never saw all the flowers that have sprung up since.

> *The garden should be an integral part of the home, like the living room. It is not some external feature.*

Objection: "But Hellen went out with Jurgen yesterday . . ."

The nursing home may have a garden, but the home's personnel often come up with all kinds of explanations for why a resident has not been outside today, such as, "Oh, she went out yesterday." Asked if a resident has not been outside today is because he or she does not like flowers or sunshine, the staff will respond that they can't just "step out" with a resident. But the notion we are "stepping out" is the problem. The garden should be an integral part of the home, like the living room. It is not some external feature.

Naturally, it takes careful planning to use the garden on a daily basis. It has to be part of the routine of the care home. First and foremost, it should be seen as an opportunity for the individual resident to get some physical exercise, according to their abilities and needs. Some will love tending the roses, some will enjoy harvesting tomatoes, and others like to help plant, pull weeds, or feed the animals if there are animals at the home. Many will just enjoy walking around the garden and sitting in it.

Admittedly, it can be challenging to get all the residents dressed and out the door at the same time. A resident with dementia may forget they were on their way out and start taking their jacket off, and then we will have to help them put it back on; this may happen a couple of times. If these types of hindrances cause too much struggle, care home staff could just aim for a smaller group of three or four residents at a time. Whatever the plan, it is important always to think ahead; think *constant care*. Get the jackets ready, make all the necessary arrangements in advance. Otherwise, it is easy to find going outside simply impossible and give up. However, if you get more experienced with the process and go outside with a few residents on a daily basis, you will gradually make it outside with everyone at once. Just try it and see how your feelings about taking the residents out can change!

Another classic reason people give for staying inside is that not all residents like going outside. The fact that a couple of them do not like a little cold wind on their face is not a strong enough argument for never letting them get some fresh air.

Summary

Saying "hello" to the outside world, for even a brief moment, is vital. The truth is, trips outside, whether to the garden at the home or to a nearby forest or nature trail, are beneficial for both the residents and the employees. It does us all good to get a little air and light, and being out in nature can remind our residents, and ourselves, of our connectedness to something greater than ourselves. I am not sure why so many people assume that working at a nursing home means staying indoors. Let people go outside; it is good for all of us.

———— • ◆ • ————

Questions for Reflection

1. Consider the story of the "stress garden" as told by a relative. Are there issues in your care home that are similarly stuck because, for instance, it is unclear who has responsibility for addressing a problem? How would you work with these issues?

2. Describe your care home's approach to incorporating time outdoors for residents. How does your approach differ from that described in this chapter?

3. Make a list of sources of nature near your care home. These could include city parks or gardens, state or national forests, and so on. List the logistical steps needed to take a group of residents out to one of these locations. What would you need to bring? Who would need to be involved?

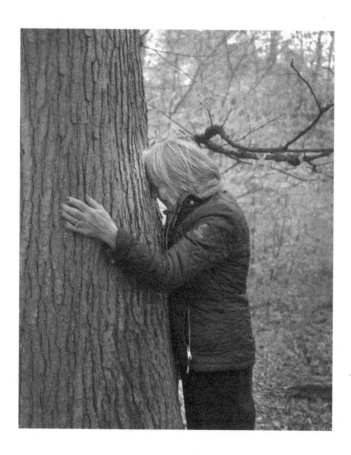

13

—◆—

Nourishing Body
and Mind

IMAGINE YOU ARE HIKING IN the desert. You are tired and worn out because you have been walking for a long time. You are nearly out of water, but you continue your journey toward an unknown destination. Right when you are on the brink of collapse, you see something on the horizon: an oasis. With your last ounce of strength, you drag yourself over to what turns out to be a lush, green area with nice people who welcome you with palm fans, cold drinks, and delicious food. You have survived. This kind of "care oasis" is what I envisioned for Dagmarsminde.

Most people coming here, like those who find themselves at any nursing home, have experienced great hardship. They may not have been cared for properly or even had enough to eat and drink. At some point, they could not decide what to buy at the supermarket, they had difficulty cooking meals, or they simply forgot to eat.

Dagmarsminde is the oasis they finally arrive at, physically and mentally exhausted. We are here to nourish them. New residents usually need to put on some pounds, having lost so much weight from an inadequate and unbalanced diet. They have not had enough fluids, which makes them confused and less resilient to exterior stimuli—already a challenge for people with dementia. The right nutrition enables a person to develop. When a resident arrives, our primary focus is ensuring they get nutrient-rich food and plenty of fluids.

Dinner Is Served at the Care Oasis

Residents continually need to be offered water, fruit juice, or maybe a cup of hot cocoa or milk. We need to restore their fluid balance so their bodies can become more resilient. This is part of laying the groundwork for good overall health.

Our bodies need nutritional balance and equilibrium, and for some new residents that means relearning how to eat. We often discover that many of them have had a poor diet for a very long time. If they have come from another nursing home, the menu was likely not only unvaried, but it was also often machine blended. They have get used to eating regular food again, which they do with great enthusiasm as their gastrointestinal system gets back on track.

Many of our new care home residents take laxatives, but these medications quickly become unnecessary once they begin consuming a varied diet, drinking plenty of fluids, and getting more exercise. We keep a fluids chart for those who tend not to drink enough, mostly to remind ourselves to keep an eye on their intake. Meanwhile, we try to figure out what each resident enjoys drinking. For example, we have a woman who absolutely will not touch water. She gets soda, juice, and milk.

Community Dining

We always eat together. The most basic reason for doing this is that sharing a meal usually means eating more. Also, when we sit around the table together, we talk about the food, and we see everyone's reaction. Sharing a meal together at the table instills a sense of familiarity and routine, and our residents enjoy it. It is important to note that we are very careful to make sure that everyone's hands are clean—both residents and staff—and all surfaces are cleaned and disinfected before we sit down.

The food needs to be appealing and nicely served. For a while, we served everyone from a platter on the table. But we found that did not work very well because most of the residents insisted on getting served first. They can get impatient, as if sitting on pins and needles, and continuously ask, "When are we going to eat?" People with dementia have a hard time with delayed gratification. Therefore, it works better when we arrange the food on the plates beforehand, or when we walk around the table with a beautifully arranged platter, serving them individually. We need peace and quiet around the table as soon as possible after people are seated so that everyone can become happily engrossed in the meal. We serve dinner restaurant-style, meaning the residents sit down to a neatly set table while food is prepared in the kitchen and then brought out to them.

We have more or less divided the residents into two groups, but the tables are close enough for us to feel connected as a group. The staff are strategically placed to ensure peace and order, in case anyone gets restless and decides to stand up. From time to time, arguments may arise or a resident may make unacceptable comments about the way someone else eats. One staff member takes on the task of serving the food and then sits down to eat with the rest of the people at the table. As much as possible, the staff try to avoid getting up for things throughout the meal. They sit down and eat along with the group, helping residents as needed along the way. The staff always sit with residents on both sides of them, particularly the ones who need help eating. Only very rarely do we actually have to feed the residents, but a bit of coaxing or coaching is often necessary.

In general, residents have their own designated seats at the table. We set the table with place cards. We do this partly so that residents can spot their names and partly to avoid problems at the table. Seeing their name reassures them that they are sitting in the right place. Once in a while, we have to switch people around because of tensions or anxieties that arise at times between residents. One person might be fiddling with a napkin, or another does not have a good grasp on his or her fork—which then irritates whoever is sitting across the table. The group dynamics are constantly changing, and getting the seating to work can sometimes be a leap of faith. It takes time, and it is always an ongoing discussion between the staff. Seating plans are continually adjusted, especially when there are new residents at the table. Yet even though most of the residents have little to no filter when it comes to speaking to others, there is generally a level of respect and politeness around the table. We make it work. No one ever eats alone in their room.

Life at Our Home

A new resident moved in and we were struggling to find the right place for her at the table. No matter where we sat her, she would get up and walk away after a couple of bites, going to the parking lot, the sofa area, down the hall, or to our shared resting area. There wasn't really any pattern to it, just that she kept getting up. The staff repeatedly walked after her, saying, "Come back Mary, we're still eating." She would go back to the table, sit down and eat for a minute, and get up again. We put our heads together to figure out why our seating plan wasn't working for Mary. It made no difference whether or not one of us sat next to her during the meal.

One day, a staff member remembered that her husband had told us that Mary had always loved inviting people over for dinner and preparing welcome drinks, snacks, full-course dinners, and cocktails. She would dress the part and was truly in her element. From then on, before every meal, a staff member would follow Mary to the bathroom and help fix her hair and put on lipstick and perfume. Then they would go to the table and fold napkins together, set the table, and pour water for everyone. The staff worker divided Mary's food into separate dishes, served on little platters around Mary's empty plate. Mary then sat down and served herself from the different dishes, and ate, occasionally looking up at the rest of us to propose a toast. She has been present for the entire meal ever since.

Eating together also allows us to keep a close watch on how much each resident is actually consuming. The staff members have a good eye for seeing if someone could use a few more bites. Perhaps there is a reason why a resident has left food on his or her plate. A bit of meat might have snuck under the lettuce and the resident did not notice there was any left, or the person might simply believe he or she has already eaten it. Therefore, we constantly have to observe what they have on their plates and make sure they finish everything. The residents may not necessarily be full just because they have stopped eating.

We also have to ensure that individual residents get down to business when they sit down to eat. Some of them do not entirely understand that the food on their plate is theirs, or what to do with it. We have to help them understand: "Right now we are sitting and eating . . . may I hold your fork for you? I'll help you taste some of this. . ." We cannot just sit down across from a resident and think they will notice that we are eating and realize they should start eating, too. We often have to work hard to ensure that the residents get enough to eat. We provide staff meals free of charge every time they eat with us, but they earn every bit of it.

Our goal is for eating to be a sensory experience— not just the act of consuming nutrients.

Ingredients

At Dagmarsminde, the food we serve is made of quality ingredients. Our goal is for eating to be a sensory experience, not just the act of consuming nutrients. Breakfast consists of fresh home-baked bread or rolls, which someone from the overnight team bakes early in the morning. It is a naturally leavened sourdough that is easy to prepare. It simply has to be taken out of the fridge, shaped, and put into the oven.

We make oatmeal for those who like it, and we offer both plain and flavored varieties of both regular and Greek yogurt, served with syrup and fruit. We also make scrambled eggs for those who like them. In addition, we include butter, cheese, and marmalade. For drinks we serve coffee, tea, water, and different juices. Platters with organic fruit, which we slice early in the morning, are always nearby throughout the home. We replenish these throughout the day so that residents can have some fruit when they wish. If a resident wants fruit on top of his or her oatmeal, a staff member adds it from these platters.

Our lunches are not lavish, but they are not unambitious either. Whatever we serve needs to be appetizing to the residents. Our lunches remind them of the open-faced sandwiches they ate in their youth, when they were active and healthy. We have different toppings to choose from—for instance, an exciting cheese, dark or white bread, and lettuce and other vegetables. We offer different toppings for the sandwiches every day, even if residents do not remember what they had yesterday. No one wants the same old piece of ham every day. The food we serve is another way of showing how we value the residents.

We serve water at every meal. This might seem a little unusual, but it is clean and clear, and it cleanses the body better than anything else. We add some lemon and orange slices for a hint of sweet or sour. But the main flavors come from the food.

As mentioned in Chapter 9, members of our overnight team are responsible for mixing the cake batter during their shift, so that the day team can pop it in the oven while the residents are taking their noontime nap. This way, they awaken to the scent of home-baked cake, which we then serve with our afternoon coffee or tea. The cakes are popular. There is even a kind of competition among the staff, so that sometimes the baked sweets look like something from a central Copenhagen confectioner.

Two times a week, we have our English-inspired high tea, both to add a little variety and also to ensure that the residents do not eat cake every single afternoon. In this way, our sweet goodies remain a novelty. One high tea may consist of little sandwiches with smoked salmon and avocado and another, ham and cucumber. Our staff carefully place all the little sandwich rectangles on a stand—exactly as is done in a traditional London hotel.

The meal the residents look forward to the most is dinner. The chef who prepares our food is very committed and has his own catering company. He prepares the food in his kitchen and sends it over; all we have to do is heat it up when it arrives. The food he prepares varies from day to day but it always includes three or four components that are easy to prepare. He reinvents traditional dishes—some of them found in centuries-old cookbooks—and then adds his own twist, borne of his love for the ingredients and for the people who will eat his food. It perfectly suits our fundamental values. The residents get to enjoy some traditional Danish dishes, which they recognize from their lives, and our chef makes sure to preserve the original flavors.

At other times, the meals are more exotic, and often something our residents have never heard of. It can be a lot of fun. They are curious and enthusiastic: "What in the world is that?" For example, we recently had the pleasure of tasting picadillo, which is a traditional South American dish with coriander, roasted tomatoes, vegetables, and marinated cucumber. Once, we had a lunch with sausages stuffed with French morels or chanterelles on a bed of chickweed and cress, which our chef picks in the forests south of Copenhagen. We have enjoyed pesto made with wild ramsons and topped with gooseberry preserve and Parmesan cheese, and American pineapple–rum pie. Another day, we might have something as ordinary to Danish people as tartlets or baked lingcod with onion cress and a mussel sauce with salted lemons, or lamb sweetbreads or chicken breasts with a velouté sauce and chervil. An assortment of different foods and flavors can help stimulate the residents' curiosity. It can also restore their faith that life still has a lot to offer.

We always eat our desserts in front of the television. It gives residents an opportunity to get up and walk around a little before they sit down on the sofa and watch the daily news. Dessert is often simple, but not just pudding or layer cake. We want our desserts to be as good as something we might find at a restaurant, and they are different every day. We might have burnt figs with vanilla ice cream or baked bananas. The latter probably sounds a little weird, but we actually had that once; it was a whole banana, with a slit for a dash of rum. A number of the residents laughed out loud and asked, "What's that supposed to be?" But it was truly delicious. Basically, we like to surprise our residents with the food.

Alcohol

We seldom serve alcohol because it is not generally good for people with dementia. Alcohol plays havoc on their minds, just as it does our own. But for someone with dementia, the effect is much worse, and they also cannot handle a hangover. Uneasiness, anxiety, headaches, and nausea are pure misery for a person who does not understand why they are suffering. We are open to the occasional small glass of something, but if we are serving wine at a celebration or during dinner in the weekends, it is usually a good, non-alcoholic wine that our local wine merchant has recommended for our residents. They drink it with pleasure, and might even let us know when they think they have reached their limit.

The Norm:
"Five o'clock is for feedings and fruit juice."

At many nursing homes, food is delivered in warm boxes from a central kitchen. Others are equipped with a large kitchen of their own. In either case, the food has to be transported to all the different floors and, hopefully, kept warm along the way. Staff members can be seen rolling the meals down the halls in big, heated, canteen-looking carts, like a feeding trough. The staff, covered in plastic aprons, will stand by the metal carts and ladle some thick brown sauce onto the mashed potatoes and sausage for each resident.

The weaker residents are often fed first. Many are characterized as "nibblers." In any case, their food is blended and served in the plastic container. The rationale may be something like, "Doris doesn't know the difference." Afterward, she is rolled over next to a window, where she sits and stares, with her back to the other residents. This way, no one has to see that she has spilled food on herself.

Plop, plop. Dinner's served for the rest of the residents—usually in their rooms, alone, but otherwise in a cafeteria or group dining area. Whatever the setting, the staff typically serve something along the lines of mashed potatoes coated in thick, lukewarm sauce; a dry, waxen sausage; and the obligatory nondescript fruit juice to wash it all down. During group dining, the staff member just moves down the rows, dropping food onto the residents' plates and looking for a place to sit, hopefully next to a fellow staff member. No one needs to help the residents if some food does not make it into their mouths because the residents have clothing protectors made of paper and plastic strung around their necks. These make them look like old babies with huge bibs, which reflects what the staff and management really think of the elderly residents: They're not normal adults anymore; they eat like babies.

Is the dining situation cozy, is it dignified, is the food nutritious and tasty? These questions are rarely asked. Even if residents and their relatives share their opinions about the mealtime horror scenarios, I suspect these comments are brushed off as empty complaints, dismissed with the useless response: "I hear what you're saying." But no action is taken to improve things.

The staff do not usually touch the food themselves, which I understand. Yet despite the depressing atmosphere I have described, these meals represent the day's main "activity" at many care homes. There is seldom anything else happening, so breakfast, lunch, and dinner more or less represent the only communal events. Not only is the mood of mealtimes unnatural and alienating, but getting the residents fed is just another task that needs completing before the staff get to go home, into the real world, where people enjoy food and have a hankering for something other than fruit juice. In reality, there is also another reason for the indifference toward meals. Some nursing homes serve cold food for dinner, which allows them to cut down on staff during those hours.

Here is the perspective of a woman whose mother was a resident in one of these nursing homes:

> Whenever I visited my mom in the evenings, I often saw the staff preparing sandwiches for the residents. Afterward, they sat them around a table with their food in front of them. While the residents ate, the staff stood leaning against the back table, impatiently glaring at them. I don't ever remember seeing the evening staff sitting down at the table with them. On the contrary, I actually saw staff tapping on the table's metal surface, as though signaling, "Hurry up and chew, so we can get you to bed." Later, I often saw the same personnel, after all the residents were put to bed, sitting in the shared living room in front of the TV, eating their own food. They didn't feel like eating with the residents. They preferred to first put them down for the night, so they could relax and eat their own food. At least that was the feeling in the pit of my stomach when I later drove home.

When you hear these kinds of stories from relatives, you get a sense of how little interest there is in creating a sense of community around the food. There is no "you and I are eating together now."

In these situations, the staff do not see with their own eyes how much the residents are consuming. Some residents, who do not eat at the table, are left alone in their room eating from a plastic tray. No one has a clue what or how much they are drinking and eating. They often leave food on their plate, resulting in a considerable amount of food waste. The residents who need to be fed by hand are treated even worse. It takes an incredible amount of awareness and focus to assist a resident to eat. But after a couple of hasty attempts, their meal can end almost before it has even begun. The leftover scraps are heaped together into one big mixed mouthful and forced down their throat, without any consideration for how it must feel to be fed this mysterious concoction. When the residents are unsurprisingly found to be malnourished, the nursing home will hire a dietician to fix the problem that should not have existed in the first place.

> When the residents feel happy and comfortable eating, they become healthier and more resistant to illness and injury.

Objection:
"But there's nothing wrong with our sausage."

Every time I talk about the food at nursing homes, the response I get is that my criticisms are not valid. I am sure there are the exceptional care homes with an inspiring meal plan and zero problems with malnutrition or undernourishment. More likely, the objectors do not want to face any criticism and are therefore defensive. They put up a false front and assert, "We have a good care home, and the food is fine." People in an unhealthy system will cover their ears and accept the low standards, and then they create their own rationalization that there is not anything wrong with the food. Whatever the response, I encourage everyone who works in a care home to take a fresh look at the food and what happens at mealtime, and to consider whether residents might feel better if nourished differently.

Summary

Good nutrition is not just about serving fresh, healthy food. It is about how well the food—and the way it is served—nourishes the individual residents, stimulates their senses, and engages them. Most importantly, the food should make them want more to help avoid undernourishment. When the residents feel happy and comfortable eating, they become healthier and more resistant to illness and injury. That is the main reason to serve delicious and inspiring food, and it is why we eat it ourselves, together with the residents. It feels so good to sit down to a good meal in the company of people you can trust. When you are done eating, you are nourished in both body and spirit; you have reached your care oasis. Why would we not want to provide that experience for the people in our care?

———————◆——————

Questions for Reflection

1. The chef who cooks for Dagmarsminde seems to take pride in providing high-quality, delicious food to the residents. Do you think this situation is particular to this care home or can you think of strategies for providing this level of nourishment to the people in your care home?

2. Do you agree with the author's conviction that people should never eat by themselves in their rooms, but should eat as part of a community in a shared dining room? Why or why not?

3. If your care home is not in the position to transform its nutrition program to the one described in this chapter, what are some practices that can be put in place to make eating "a sensory experience—not just the act of consuming nutrients"?

14

———— •◆• ————

Continuing Family
Traditions

ANYONE WHO ENJOYS CHRISTMASTIME, WITH all its traditions, knows the feeling: "Look, aren't those grandmother's glass ornaments on the tree? And the elves over there—we made those when we were kids . . ." Sweet memories come back to you as you decorate the tree, hang up the Advent wreath, and put candles in the windows. You may experience warmth and comfort, awash in feelings from "the good old times." Most people have experienced this kind of feeling, no matter what religion or tradition they follow.

In our Danish care home, we take the memories and the symbolism seriously, especially when we decorate for Christmas. We hang an Advent wreath from the ceiling, with red ribbon and real candles. We celebrate each Sunday in Advent and invite our residents' families to join us for freshly baked Danish doughnuts, non-alcoholic mulled wine, and hot chocolate. We provide presents, sorted into the appropriate age groups, for the children who come with their parents. We sing the old familiar hymns during our Christmas service. Everyone, including staff and residents, contributes ideas and items they remember from their own family traditions so that the entire month of December is one long "trip to Grandmother's." The whole house is decorated with elves, Christmas lights, little nativity scenes, and ornaments. Paper hearts appear in the windows, and we sing carols. We give every resident an inexpensive, personal gift—perhaps a nice barrette or a pair of warm socks.

At the stroke of 5:00 p.m. on Christmas Eve, all of us at Dagmarsminde gather for a little glass of port wine or fruit juice and make a toast. The table is set to perfection with white tablecloths and beautiful flower decorations. We eat duck, roast pork with crackling, and Danish rice pudding. As is tradition in Denmark, inside the pudding we hide a single whole almond, and whoever "wins" it usually receives a nice box of chocolates. This tradition of celebrating Christmas is a fundamental part of our lives and of the residents' lives, so it has a presence in our care home. The same is true of other life-affirming traditions and rites. If you have lived your whole life with family and friends with whom you have celebrated birthdays, Christmas, Easter, and other holidays and special occasions, it is not surprising that these celebrations are an important part of who you are. These traditions are something people take with them, wherever they go—even when they move into a nursing home.

> By observing these special occasions, we honor and respect the past lives of individual residents.

A resident might always have associated Easter with his or her family's fine porcelain eggs hanging on blossoming spring branches in a vase in their living room. Maybe there was a very specific order for how things were done on Christmas Eve, including when the tree was decorated with the ornaments. These kinds of rituals get passed down for generations and are important for everyone, which is why we emphasize them; they need to continue to the extent possible. By observing these

Life at Our Home

Anna was a resident who, in addition to dementia, also had Parkinson's disease. She was the kind of person who always participated and was always seeking company, but on Christmas Eve she suddenly did not want to join us in our shared living space. She passed the whole day in her room, even though we tried all sorts of things to reawaken her enthusiasm. We talked to her about what kind of nice dress and jewelry she would wear when her husband came for Christmas. But she remained closed off and sad. A staff member sat down next to her and asked, "What do you usually do when your family is sitting down for Christmas dinner?" Due to Parkinson's, her speech was staccato, with only one word at a time, but the staff member understood that Anna's role had been to welcome everyone to the table and tell about the food before people were seated. "Well, that's your job here too!" the staff member told her.

When all the residents and some of their relatives were heading to the table, the staff member tapped her glass and asked for everyone's attention. She presented Anna and asked them to listen to what she had to say before they sat down. Anna got up, and without any hesitation, welcomed them and presented the courses, which she said she had made, and which were also quite different from our meal that evening. But no one gave it a second thought. Glowing with pride, she lit up the room.

special occasions, we honor and respect the past lives of individual residents. In Denmark, we not only celebrate Easter and Christmas, but also the Royal birthdays, which we also make a big deal out of at the care home. Your country likely has similar traditions—for instance, Independence Day or Thanksgiving in the United States. These traditions, if they were observed in youth, remain deep in the memory, even when a person has dementia.

Even when residents forget their own birthdays, it is important that we remember it for them—and that we make their day as special as possible. You see, they have not forgotten the feeling of being celebrated. Resident birthdays are always a grand occasion at Dagmarsminde. We celebrate the individual from morning to night. We raise the flag in our garden. We wake up the birthday boy or girl with flags and a song, and have home-baked cinnamon rolls, presents, candles, and flowers at our breakfast table. We always have a gift for the resident, which he or she can open at the table. We sing "Happy Birthday," often several times a day. In the afternoon, the person's family comes for a visit, and then we have coffee and traditional Danish layer cake. We go to great lengths to ensure the day is as festive as possible, and we do everything to make it an enjoyable day for the individual resident in particular. It is that person's very own day! The residents sense it is a day filled with happy family atmosphere. They know the rest of us at the care home are not their actual family, yet they still feel that they are among family on a day like this. It is lovely to see how much it means, that we all do so much to celebrate *them*.

Life at Our Home

It was Eric's birthday. Throughout the day, we kept reminding him and the others about our celebration because otherwise they would forget. That afternoon, we brought out the cake and placed it in front of him with lit candles. This tradition is so deeply ingrained from their childhoods that all of the residents smiled and started singing "Happy Birthday" to Eric. We always make it very clear who the birthday boy or girl is.

Eric blew out the candles with everyone around him eagerly watching, because, in Denmark, if any candles are left burning, it means the birthday person is in love with someone. But Eric blew them all out. We all clapped, and, as everyone quieted down, the woman sitting next to him said, "Oh, well, I guess we're just friends then."

The Norm:
In Want of Celebration

Many care homes operate around a cyclical calendar. Their move-in brochures or resident newsletters almost always include a description of this rotating calendar, in which one activity is highlighted each month. It might look something like this:

January: New Year's Treats for the residents, relatives, and volunteers; champagne and marzipan wreath cake

February: Shrovetide with sweet rolls and games

March: Easter lunch

April: Olympics with the visiting preschool children

May: Prayer day with warm rolls

June: Summer barbecue with fun and games in the garden

July: Staff on vacation

August: Harvest Festival

September: Memory Day with Memory Cake

October: Generation Day, when relatives of all ages are invited for cake and coffee

November: Morten's Night with roasted duck and red cabbage for dinner

December: Old-fashioned Christmas luncheon

It all looks very promising. The rotating calendar checks all the boxes. But words can sometimes be empty. What kinds of thoughts or reflections are behind those words and the calendar wheel? All too often, very little. A care home might highlight the Generation Day celebration, but why is it being celebrated—because the administration and staff want to? Or are they forced to because it is written in the calendar? Often, events like these, one per month, are just institutional initiatives rather than true celebrations; they are just a contrived attempt at manufacturing culture.

I once heard a relative saying that she had brought her daughter and grandchildren with her to the care home where her mother was staying after seeing a poster in the elevator about a Generation Day party that welcomed children, grandchildren, and great-grandchildren to the home and promised coffee, cake, and lots of fun. But when the whole family turned up that afternoon and walked down to the living room area, the staff had never heard of the event. "Try checking the second floor," a staff member told the relative. But when the family went to that floor, there was no hint of a party or celebration anywhere, and they were told to check the main hall on the first floor. There, the staff recalled hearing about it, but since no one had showed up, the plans were dropped. The relative was left crestfallen and disillusioned, with her daughter, grandchildren, and her mother. Why make the effort to post those kinds of events, when the staff did not care enough to follow through? It looked great on the calendar, and no one ever added a note that it had been cancelled.

How do you fit a life into a calendar wheel? Isn't this type of calendar just another bureaucratic document, demonstrating how the care home adheres to certain rules? Leaders in the care home can show they have thought things over, and hold it up, like a school assignment, showing they have completed it. It is a confirmation of having fulfilled expectations. Unfortunately, this confirmation becomes more important than the event itself, as in the example above. If the will and the motivation are lacking, so is the celebration.

Many care homes, in Denmark and elsewhere, have adopted an institutional culture, in which staff and administrators relate to their work in the homes as "just a job"; they are like cogs in what I have called the care factory. They do not see the care home as a *home*, so when they make the effort to decorate the place for holidays or special occasions, they do not see the need to ensure that those decorations will be meaningful to the people who live there. They relate to decorating as something extra, and not as part of the care they provide.

If you visit a normal Danish care home around Christmas, you will find that a few of the halls might be decorated, but not as one would prepare for Christmas at home. The windows and ceiling may be adorned with big plastic bulbs in repeating colors, and you might notice the same style of bulbs (from the same box) hanging on the tree in the living room. Apparently, this year someone has decided on a "blue/white" theme, like they saw at the mall. There is no hint of that authentic overlap of new and old, neat and messy, of little homemade ornaments or an array of brightly colored hearts, all of which contribute to a cozy Christmas in Danish homes. When I walk through a plastic-decorated state-run institution, I get the same feeling as when I rush through an international airport in late December. I am greeted by huge plastic bulbs and plastic trees with enormous golden ribbons on them, everything a variation of pink or purple. This kind of impersonal decoration might make sense in an airport or mall, but in one's home, part of the joy of decorations is being reminded of the people we came from, young and old, throughout the generations. "This was my grandmother's paper cone" and "that's my old aunt's Christmas star shining at top of the tree." I do not believe this sentiment is unique to Denmark. A care home's Christmas needs to have the same authentic personal touch, where everyone can contribute with their favorite decorations.

> *You might be surprised at how much fun it can be*
> *to celebrate with the people in your care.*

For many people, traditions are a big part of who they are, and residents are deeply affected when their surroundings seem indifferent. Not making a point of continuing traditions ignores the importance of touching someone's heart. At many homes, staff members are on vacation in the weeks leading up to Christmas. They take time off to enjoy their own special traditions together with their own families. We do not blame them for that, but there is no reason we cannot provide a warm holiday for the people who live in our care home.

Objection: "It will never be like home."

The reason given by many who work in care homes for not observing traditions is the difficulty of recreating the traditions of every single resident. This can be a handy excuse, conveniently giving up before they have really tried. It is important to remember, though, that celebrating a birthday or other special occasion is as meaningful for the residents as it is for the rest of us. A celebration can be an important touchstone for a person whose world feels increasingly foreign. If you care about the residents, do not allow this part of life to fall by the wayside.

You might be surprised at how much fun it can be to celebrate with the people in your care. I do not know of any staff who find it boring to celebrate a resident's birthday or do something extra special for Christmas. Staff appreciate the permission to do something creative and kind for their residents—for example, creating a merry old-fashioned Christmas atmosphere or decorating a resident's seat at the table on their birthday. This kind of activity is always very popular at Dagmarsminde. My staff practically line up to decorate the place. If I have been busy, someone on my staff will come and ask, "Hey, aren't we hanging an Advent wreath this year?"

Summary

It is up to us to help our residents feel at home and appreciated by honoring their traditions and special days. Even in more institutional settings, care staff should become familiar enough with the residents in their care to understand their traditions and what could give them joy on a particular day. Cultivating this knowledge, and caring enough to do something about it, should be second nature for anyone working in the care sector.

The more energy we put into celebrating and creating a homey atmosphere, the happier the residents and the staff become.

———•◆•———

Questions for Reflection

1. How does your care home mark residents' birthdays and other special occasions?

2. If your care home is not in the position to decorate and celebrate as fully as described here, what are some ways that celebrations might be incorporated into the program of care?

3. The author states, "You might be surprised at how much fun it can be to celebrate with the people in your care." What has been your experience celebrating with the people in your care? Describe the event as well as the feelings, both positive and negative, that arose.

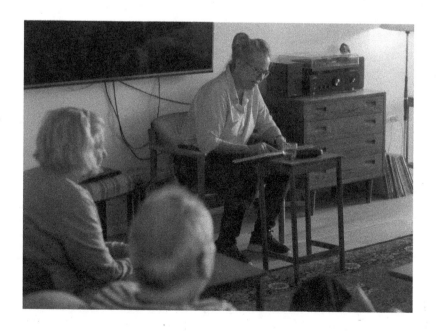

15

⋄◆⋄

Under Observation:

Looking After the Health of Our Residents

How do we keep on top of a care home resident's health? By constantly being aware of and reacting to even the smallest signs of weakening. For me, it is not complicated when we are around our residents all the time. This is one of the many rewards of a community. Keeping an eye on each resident's condition is an integral part of the work we do every single day.

Observation Processes and Staff

Naturally, we have to work on many levels in caring for our residents. We have incorporated some simple procedures to make it both easy and manageable to keep track of the individual resident's health. First, we talk face to face with the individual residents on a daily basis. Then we share our experiences and observations with the rest of the staff. We do not schedule long, daily handovers between the shifts; instead, we each keep an eye out and tell each other what we have observed during our shift.

> We have discovered that if we let individual staff members record the information in their own way, they are more likely to want to record it.

The Journal

In addition to simply talking with each other, we also keep notes on our residents in a journal. These notes, however, are not clinical or dry, as is the case in many places. At Dagmarsminde, we have discovered that if we let individual staff members record the information in their own way, they are more likely to *want* to record it. We have found that the quality of the documentation actually improves, and the health-related issues are covered in more detail. When the individual staff member is allowed to record in her own words what happened, how she responded, and the outcome—perhaps also reporting on the positive or even negative effects of one of her own initiatives—she engages wholeheartedly in the report and is personally motivated to provide the best description possible. As a result, one might say our journals are a little more poetic than is accepted at other places where the descriptions are short and clear-cut.

Our way of journaling includes more observations and details, but more importantly, this type of documentation inspires us, as we read each other's notes. A can-do spirit is encouraged by what other colleagues have accomplished, and also by the fact that they have something nice and positive to read. The journal contains much more than clinical nursing terminology; it is more of an open-ended presentation of the residents. In addition, the individual staff member also shows—and sees for herself—that as a human being, she is an integral part of the care. For example, we write "I," to encourage staff members to share their own observations and experiences with the resident, and we try to end the journal entry with the present situation. Here is a journal entry from one of our night staff:

> Karen got very sad after our evening coffee. I went to help Karen to bed, but discovered that she was sitting there on the sofa, quietly crying. I sat down next to Karen and put my arm around her. She started sobbing and continued for a long time. Karen has had a hard time finding the words for what she is

feeling, but I recall that the other day she beautifully articulated her feelings of sorrow, loss, and loneliness. At the end, Karen dried her eyes and wanted to go to bed. In the bathroom, Karen got angry that someone had forgotten to flush. "It's full of . . . piss!" Karen said angrily. I cleaned the toilet so it looked nice again. After Karen got into bed (with her long-sleeved night gown), I brought the cat that Karen loves so much. "Come to Karen," she said to the cat, happily smiling. Right now, Karen is in her bed, petting the cat, looking very content.

This more open form of journaling inspires the other staff members and makes them want to try it out themselves. Another example from our journals describes a scenario in which a resident was trying to cope with her frustration:

By lunch time, Lisbeth was very angry, wandering around the garden, scolding everyone and everything, and it was nearly impossible to talk to her or even approach her. I noticed that Lisbeth was slightly shaking, not just from anger; she was sad, with tears in her eyes. I wanted Lisbeth to eat and drink something, but she made it clear that under no circumstances was she coming back inside.

I brought some lunch out to Lisbeth and managed to get her to sit at the table under the oak tree and eat something. Lisbeth continued her tirade but let me cut her food into bite-sized pieces; I handed her a fork, which motivated her to eat half of two sandwiches and drink a glass of water. I sensed how important it was to win back her trust and show that I was on her side, an "ally," who understood how dreadful everything was and that everyone was awful, and we had to do something about it on Monday. Lisbeth gradually calmed down, and I was able to guide her back—and in we walked, arm in arm, through the living room. She felt safe again. Lisbeth let herself be led to the bathroom; back in her room, she took her long pants off by herself and allowed me to tuck her into bed, with the blinds completely closed, lying on her side with a pillow behind her back for support. I put the heavier down comforter on top of Lisbeth's own comforter. Then I sat near the headboard and rested my hand on her forehead for a little while. She fell asleep more quickly than usual, and she slept for half an hour. Lisbeth woke up happy and content, with no signs of restlessness or anger.

So how does this more narrative way of sharing important information actually help improve our residents' condition? When staff members inspire each other and are motivated to try out new initiatives, residents sense the dynamic energy and can feel encouraged to play an active role in their own development; they begin to feel healthier themselves.

The White Board

In the office at Dagmarsminde, we keep an electronic white board filled with notes about the residents' needs. Some examples of notes that might appear in the field for a given resident are the following:

- *Needs long walks in the forest*
- *Has problems swallowing, transition to soft food evaluated next week*
- *Needs to be tucked in tightly when resting*

Need for stimulation, need for rest, need for conversation—we include more than merely physical, measurable values. We record those too, but we spend most of the time on our needs-related observations. Residents' blood pressure readings, fluid levels, and other kinds of measurements are more of a journal entry than a topic for conversation.

ADCS–ADL

As I mentioned in Chapter 6, we screen our residents' skills using the American screening tool Alzheimer's Disease Cooperative Study–Activities of Daily Living (ADCS–ADL). Every other month, we tally each resident's scores and assess which areas we need to focus on. For example, a resident may seem to have become less capable of getting dressed. We consider the overall picture we have of the resident's abilities, and if we assess that there is a possibility of regaining the ability to get dressed, we decide to put our efforts into helping the person with that. Another ability is eating with a knife and fork or pouring a cup of coffee. We test and train residents' skills repeatedly, which helps us become more aware of their level of skill as well as the progress of their condition.

Staff Meeting

Once a week we have a staff meeting that lasts about an hour and a half. We review everything we know about each resident—weight, blood pressure, mental status, and abilities. Has the person become more capable or less capable at doing certain things? We cover all the residents, but delve a little deeper into the progress of one or two whom we have selected beforehand for additional review. These might be residents who recently moved in, for example, or those who have needed additional attention for a period. In these meetings, we often decide on a certain approach or way of doing things, which we then communicate to the rest of the staff.

Nurses and Doctors

Our nurses also play an important role in preventing acute conditions, hospitalizations, and physical decline. We have more trained nurses here than at most care homes, and they are not hired to sit behind a desk or be summoned only for special situations. Our nurses participate in the daily direct care like anyone else, which adds a further level of prevention. As health professionals, nurses offer a unique perspective, and on the whole they add to the well-being of our residents.

The nurses have the expertise to perform a number of clinical tasks, further ensuring the stability of our residents' health. For example, they can perform a urine culture if we suspect a urinary tract infection. This way, we can prescribe the correct antibiotics and start treatment as early as possible, which is crucial for avoiding hospitalizations due to bladder infections. People with dementia are prone to urinary tract infections because many use incontinence pads or do not wipe properly if unassisted in the bathroom. This poses a huge challenge at most care homes because the staff are not qualified to do a urine culture and have to send their urine samples to a doctor for testing, which results in delayed treatment.

So far, we have not had a single hospitalization due to a urinary tract infection. From time to time, our residents develop them, but because we check frequently and initiate treatment from the outset, they are not allowed to become as severe as they do in other care homes. In addition, we almost always accompany the residents to the bathroom and ensure that they clean themselves thoroughly afterward. For those residents who use incontinence pads, we ensure that they are not exposed to a moist pad for very long. Even for those who wear pads, we typically find only small traces of urine because we make sure the residents go to the bathroom regularly. The result is that very few of them are actually incontinent. They urinate in the toilet.

I think we prevent the majority of infections by having nurses working in our direct care. Once again, we see nursing as craft, with the nurses sharing their knowledge with the rest of the staff. Other members of the staff are also trained within the field, but the nurses have the final say on any new treatment protocols. The nurses work closely with our care work assistants; our support workers; and our brilliant, out-of-the-box–thinking, untrained co-workers. Our team consists of different health professionals and different kinds of people, providing for people with different strengths. This diversity of background is exactly what our residents need.

Once a month, our general practitioner comes for a visit. The meeting with him happens in much the same manner as our staff meeting, in which we evaluate all of the residents, one by one. With our doctor, though, our evaluation covers everything medically related, such as potential adjustments to residents' medications; blood sample results; referrals to specialists; and examinations of the residents for any clinical issues, such as back pain, coughing, or heart arrhythmias. We also consult the doctor about any residents whose chronically weak condition appears terminal. After meeting with us, the doctor makes the rounds to some of the residents; they are seen by the doctor if we feel at all concerned or have any doubts.

Life at Our Home

Life with Sarah was a ball. She was full of compliments, giving hugs as we passed, and was always dancing and singing. As time passed, she seemed tired at times, but she was still in high spirits throughout the day. Then, at a certain point within a short timeframe, we noticed several big changes. She became more introverted and it sounded forced when she tried to be funny. She seemed tense and was constantly seeking our attention. We suspected it was a urinary tract infection, a toothache, or perhaps some unpleasantry with another resident. But we were able to rule those out. We looked at every possible cause for the change in her mood. She didn't appear to be suffering physically, but in our shared discussions with her family, and in hearing their observations, we gathered that her life was nearing its natural end. As her dementia advanced, it got harder and harder for her to live up to her perception of herself as a fun-filled, energized person. Her self-understanding was facing a dramatic transformation and, on top of that, she was also very old.

We decided, with the family's acceptance, to put her previous "Pollyanna" persona behind us and to fully embrace and acknowledge the more introverted person she had become. This turned out to be a good idea because, from then on, she seemed more comfortable in her own skin, accepting she that didn't have to be entertaining all the time. The following 2 months were stable and comfortable for her. After that period, she lost her appetite and her interest in joining our different activities, and she quietly and calmly said goodbye to this world.

The Norm:
"He's just a little tired these days . . ."

We have the ability to improve a care home resident's health simply by sharpening our awareness of the person. But many care homes simply are not set up to be on the alert. We often hear the argument that this level of care is "a losing battle" for people who have dementia and are old. Many homes, at least in Denmark, do not observe their residents systematically on a daily basis.

We have to look at the whole picture of each resident in order to assess his or her state of health. If you see it as normal and acceptable to view the residents as older and having dementia—and therefore "on the way out," then you probably also think it is alright for them to be a little under the weather and depressed. This kind of thinking can be life-threatening, though, especially when everyone starts believing it. When everyone around the resident thinks this way, the resident will only get weaker and, ultimately, critically ill.

When people talk about my care home, they say, "It's easy for you—you only get healthy residents." But our residents are exactly as vulnerable as the residents at any other care home. The difference is that we make a daily effort to maintain the health of our residents, until the day they naturally decline and die. We keep an eye on them, constantly observing their condition, ensuring that they stay healthy for as long as possible. Maybe this is why they appear healthier than residents at other places. They move around and hold their head high, they laugh and engage with others, and they have a will to live.

> There are many parts of a resident's condition that cannot be measured with a medical instrument.

It is easy to keep an eye on the residents in our care. It does not necessarily need to take more time. Instead, think about how time gets used. For example, how many meetings are held on a daily basis at most care homes? The handover meetings between daytime staff and those working in the evening often use up an hour every day. Imagine if the handover only took 10 minutes, and instead the staff held an hour-long meeting once a week, where they reviewed all the residents together. Utilizing our time carefully allows more time to be available to our residents and fosters a togetherness that affords a unique insight into their condition and allows for better observation and problem solving.

Objection:
"Her blood pressure is in the journal . . ."

The general opinion among many who care for people with dementia is that the person's health is under control when the vital signs—blood pressure, weight, and temperature—are steady and within normal limits. But there are so many parts of the resident's condition that cannot be measured with a medical instrument. The person's frame of mind and will to live are crucial for maintaining their stability. These human values need to be more prominent so they are considered of equal value to blood pressure readings, dietary management, and other information. Any care home bearing this in mind will immediately make headway. By focusing on the residents' human needs, those who care for them can prevent many of the unstable conditions that commonly occur in people with dementia.

The fundamental problem is that most care homes do not have enough health professionals onsite. The majority of care home personnel are not trained in prevention and in performing the basic medical tests. Far too many older adults are unnecessarily hospitalized simply because the people caring for them are unsure how to help them and are afraid to engage with them on a human level.

Summary

Having more trained nurses working in direct care can prevent illness and treat any infections before they worsen. With these basic medical and physical aspects of health under control, staff should see the residents in their care as much more than their blood pressure and temperature readings. Working with a resident's health means seeing the whole person. Only by engaging with that whole person on a daily basis can we observe changes that will help us to determine the best possible care.

Questions for Reflection

1. Consider the method of journaling used by staff at Dagmarsminde. Does your care home record resident progress in a similar way? How does your current method differ?

2. Recall the last time you or your staff noticed a dramatic change in a resident, similar to the resident who was having new difficulty getting dressed, or Sarah, whose personality began to change. How was that change addressed? Was the outcome satisfactory? Why or why not?

3. Are there processes described in this chapter that could be helpful to implement in your care home? If so, list the steps that might be involved to make that happen.

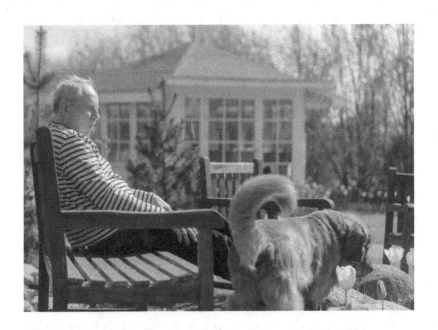

PART TWO

The Weakening Phase

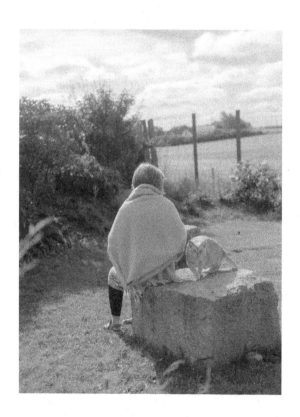

16

◦ ◆ ◦

Swallowing Problems

When Eating Solid Foods Becomes Difficult

THE WEAKENING PHASE BEGINS WHEN a resident with dementia approaches the final phase of illness and begins showing signs of approaching the end of life. The first of these signs is difficulty swallowing regular food. At this point, the resident's motor skills are beginning to decline. It is hard for them to walk and difficult for them to comprehend the connection between bringing the fork up to their mouth and getting something to eat. This tells us they are entering the weakening phase. It is the same for almost everyone with dementia; once we detect an issue with swallowing, we realize what is happening.

Coughing

The weakening phase almost always starts with coughing. The resident starts coughing after meals, for example, if the food—such as rye bread, granola, or rolls—has small crumbs that easily get stuck in the throat. It's a kind of tickle, as if something is irritating the throat, and leads to a coughing fit. During this phase, though, the coughing is unproductive because the resident no longer has the capacity to finish the cough. We hear them constantly clearing their throat, along with a kind of "brassy" high-pitched cough. The resident takes a long time to swallow and might even store a bit of fluid and food in the mouth because he or she does not understand where the food is supposed to go.

Coughing is a common sign that the dementia has advanced to the point at which the person's ability to eat is affected. The weakness in the muscles of the person's mouth impacts his or her swallowing and the esophagus; besides this, the resident no longer senses the food in his or her mouth. Continuing to give the person regular food at this point will not help; it will only worsen the coughing. He or she might start drooling or spitting the food out. As the disease advances, other foods—not just dry bread, salad, and so on—can irritate the throat. Even blended foods can lead to serious coughing fits. At the very end, the resident is not able to swallow any liquids either.

Life at Our Home

We were surprised during dinner one day to hear Esther coughing, especially because the meal was a creamy Italian pasta dish that shouldn't have caused any swallowing issues. But the same thing happened the next morning with her yogurt. Her coughing only worsened when she took a sip of orange juice. Many hours later, as we walked with her around the garden, we could still hear how the coughing had affected her breathing. By the following meal, we concluded that Esther had developed swallowing problems and would require closer attention. From that point on, we made sure there wasn't anything in her food that could irritate her throat. We also started adding an amylase-resistant thickener to her liquids. Unfortunately, we had to hold back the orange juice she so loved. Instead, we made her iced coffee with syrup in the mornings. Her coughing stopped, but if we tried giving her a little salad or something similar, her cough quickly returned. Esther's food requirements had clearly changed, and we knew the staff were going to have to be extra creative when preparing her meals.

Changes in Food and Eating

In order to avoid complications, such as gagging or pneumonia, we have to react as soon as the swallowing difficulties arise. After only a few days of observing the symptoms, we decide to switch to softer foods. Starting out, we avoid rye bread, crisp breads, and anything in this category. As the resident's condition progresses, we will only give the person softer foods, such as yogurt or soft white bread in the morning. After that, the resident's food is usually pureed.

We always try to give the resident with swallowing difficulties the same food as the rest of us, and while we have to puree theirs, we still make sure it tastes good. It has to feel like real food. Of course, eating a potato pureed with meat and vegetables will never feel as normal as eating it whole, but the resident gets something that looks and tastes similar. At times, we run into the problem that some meals are not suited for blending; in that case, we buy special meals for the residents with swallowing difficulties. These might include some good soups that we can heat up. The person in this phase may also be more interested in vanilla ice cream.

At the first sign that a resident is having trouble swallowing, we make sure to explain to the relatives what is happening.

Some of the larger care homes have an even greater ability to prepare and serve soft foods. There are no limits to what they can do to make the often aesthetically challenging food look normal. We can also learn from some places within the hospital sector that are developing and refining this type of food. Otherwise, I recommend getting inspiration from other places such as Japan and the United States, where the care sectors are making great strides with making softened food look more appealing, using coloring agents and shapes to make it look more like regular food.

The initial swallowing problems gradually worsen, and this phase can stretch over a long time—often several months. At the first sign that a resident is having trouble swallowing, we make sure to explain to the relatives what is happening. They need to know why we are suddenly serving their loved one blended food. We also talk about it with the residents themselves, but they usually do not understand the connection. It is very important that the relatives do not misinterpret our actions. It is futile for them to bring all sorts of edible treats for their loved one when they visit; often they want to do this because they worry that the blended food is insufficient, or they just want their loved one to have something that tastes good. However, a tiny piece of chocolate can cause a lot of grief.

When we eat together, the resident with swallowing difficulties sits at the table with the rest of us. We make sure a staff member is keeping a close watch on whether the resident is swallowing the food with no issues. Without close attention, food or drink can get stuck in the cavity of the resident's mouth. From the outside, it may seem that the resident is swallowing, but he or she may not follow through with that. If we are not alert, there could still be something in the mouth that can quickly go down the wrong way if the person starts drifting off. Therefore, it is important that whoever is sitting next to the person tells him or her plainly, "It's time to swallow" or "Drink," after every mouthful.

We constantly try to stimulate the resident in some way, so he or she remembers to swallow correctly. We might touch the side of his or mouth, for example. We pay attention to the muscles in the throat, looking to see if the food and fluids are passing through. If the resident happens to inhale any food particles instead of swallowing them, it can cause a type of pneumonia that is difficult to treat with penicillin. It is also important to consider that swallowing problems often lead to poor oral hygiene, which adds the potential complication of respiratory tract infections.

> *Taking time to slow down can be critical to
> maintaining the resident's quality of life.*

Something else to watch out for in residents with advanced dementia in the weakening phase is a tendency to grab anything on the table and put it in their mouth. Their cognitive functions may be so impaired that they do not understand that some things on the table are not meant to be eaten—such as flowers, napkins, and so on. This is why it is not enough to leave food in front of them and let them eat or drink on their own. You constantly have to watch them. These residents may also develop an oral fixation, perhaps from missing the sensation of chewing and feeling different textures in their mouth, which may lead to a preoccupation with putting whatever is right in front of them in their mouth. For example, one of our residents started chewing on her barrette.

Once again, taking time to slow down can be critical to maintaining the resident's quality of life. We try not to put pressure on a resident who is not swallowing properly, especially if he or she is eating too fast. Sometimes we can mitigate swallowing problems by sitting with the resident at the table for a little while, allowing him or her to begin eating or drinking before the others join us at the table. It can also help to work with very small portions. My advice, always: Take your time.

The Norm:
Hurried Meals

Pneumonia is often the real cause behind the "natural" deaths of many older adults. Unfortunately, it still is not standard practice at Danish care homes to investigate the causes of pneumonia. Staff members may be unaware of the initial signs that the resident has reached the onset of the weakening phase. A few coughs after meals does not usually raise any concern; in fact, the staff may be more alarmed if the resident were not ailing in some way. A cough may be seen as just a cough. The reason for the coughing is considered to be of little consequence. At some point, staff may realize the ongoing cough is in fact due to swallowing problems and the onset of the weakening phase, but they may continue giving the person solid food, as though nothing has changed. They do not set aside more time to care for the resident. They do not offer a softer diet or the necessary time and calm to allow the resident to swallow properly.

For the resident with swallowing problems, a hastened meal can easily lead to choking, which is often followed by pneumonia and hospitalizations. Pneumonia is one of the most widespread reasons for hospitalizations of older care home residents. Often, the person hospitalized for pneumonia dies of so-called "natural causes."

All of these hospitalizations followed by death are an unnecessary and easily avoided expense. More importantly, this is an undignified way for a person to end their days. I am convinced that many of the hospitalizations due to pneumonia are partly the result of staff members taking too long to discover a resident's problems with swallowing. They simply are not paying attention to how a resident is eating—most often because they do not eat with the residents. Residents with swallowing problems are often bedridden, so staff members may bring the food to their room intending to help them eat, but that help ends up being brief because they have to hurry out for other tasks.

The resident's pneumonia, malnourishment, and fluid imbalance can go undetected for too long. The resident also lacks the basic fundamental daily stimulation of eating and drinking. Very soon, he or she no longer has the strength to cough and starts gasping for air with a slight rattle at the end. The person is simultaneously hungry, thirsty, and frail—and does not understand what is happening. But it does not have to be like this.

At Dagmarsminde, we have yet to see a resident die of pneumonia. When our residents die, they die here with us, at

the care home, and only because they no longer have the will
to endure. They are sated by life, as I discuss in Chapter 17.
In the final phase of dementia, they completely stop eating and
drinking, and it is completely natural.

Objection:
"Anyone have time to go feed Kirsten?"

Why should it pose such a huge problem for a staff member
to take time out to sit with someone who has problems swallowing food? Apparently for many care homes in Denmark and
elsewhere, the issue is complicated. When looking at the causes
of death for care home residents, most of them are due to poor
nutrition, fluid imbalance, respiratory issues, dizziness, or falling. I think the reality is that many of these places see it as
a chore to have to feed residents. In fact, it is a slow, quiet,
and somewhat monotonous task. The staff members who pride
themselves on doing these kinds of basic tasks are few and far
between.

The staff at care homes can convince themselves they do
not have the time or resources to guide and support the resident with reminders to swallow. The other challenging aspect,
as mentioned previously, is that at this stage of the disease the
resident may be so frail that he or she is mainly bedridden,
perhaps tucked away in a corner of the care home, because it
is easier to keep the person "safe" that way. It is an oppressive
form of care.

What usually happens in the end is that no one takes time
out of their busy schedule to go feed the resident. They lose
track, rushing from one task to the next, and it can feel as
though there is no room for the onerous task of helping a resident with swallowing problems get anything to eat. Imagine if
the resident were helped out of bed and joined the rest in the
living room. There, he or she would automatically be seen, not
forgotten. The staff could consider how to manage their time
for that person's benefit. That is exactly what the person needs.

Summary

The first sign that a person is entering the weakening phase of dementia toward the end of life is difficulty swallowing, often signaled by a cough that occurs after eating. It is important to notice these problems in time to address them with soft or pureed food, not only to prevent the resident from choking or developing pneumonia from food aspiration, but also to alert the relatives of the situation so that they do not bring solid food for their loved ones to enjoy. Equally critical to noticing these problems before it is too late is spending time eating with residents, or at least observing them carefully as they eat. Slowing down can provide both a way to discover the problem and a means for working with it.

———•◆•———

Questions for Reflection

1. The author points to undetected or unaddressed swallowing problems as a primary cause of pneumonia in older adults with dementia. Explain why you agree or disagree with this argument.

2. Consider how the staff at your organization manage swallowing difficulties that arise in the late stage of dementia. Are these problems noticed early enough to prevent choking incidents, pneumonia, or hospitalization? If not, what changes would help?

3. The author makes the point in different ways throughout the book that "Taking time to slow down can be critical to maintaining the resident's quality of life." Do you agree with this advice? Consider some ways that staff members at your organization might be encouraged, or allowed, to slow down.

17

◦◆◦

Approaching the
End of Life

IT IS COMPLETELY NORMAL THAT people who have lived for many years with dementia, or any condition of decline, should at some point feel finished with life and want peace. In Chapter 16, I described how swallowing difficulties are often among the first noticeable signs of physical decline due to dementia. In this chapter, I take a closer look at how we, as care staff, can determine when a person has lost his or her *appetite for life*.

Common Signs of Decline

In general, there are a number of signs that can reveal a resident is on the way toward the final phase. Following are some of these signs:

- Constant fatigue; increase in sleeping
- Refusal of and physically turning away from offers of food and liquids
- Introversion, both physically and socially
- Less eye contact; eyes often closed in social situations
- General avoidance of social situations

- Episodes of not fully recovering from colds, bladder infections, or other infections
- Inability to regain strength after hospitalizations and operations

We often observe how the resident starts to withdraw. The interest he or she once had in participating in the care home's shared activities gradually diminishes. Likewise, the person shows no interest when invited to do something alone with us. The resident becomes strangely detached, although it is difficult to ascertain the exact reason why. It might not even be anything specific. We see the resident losing interest in the world around him or her, from the moment of waking until going to bed. It is not because of anger or sadness. The person's distant manner could also be seen as indifference or a kind of resolve. You can tell by the look on the person's face; it takes a lot to bring out even a tiny smile, and it is almost impossible to get people to laugh during this phase. It is as though the resident is somewhere else entirely.

The resident loses all interest in eating and drinking. Both the mental and physical appetite disappears. At the beginning, we often hear the resident saying he or she has no desire or need for regular food. We might be able to tempt the person with sweet foods because the taste for sweetness tends to last a little longer than the other tastes. For a little while, the resident subsists on cake, flavored yogurts, ice cream, and the like. But even so, the person does not eat very much of it, and eats almost mechanically, without interest. By this point, swallowing issues have usually begun as well.

If the transformation is sudden, and continues, it is usually a sign that the resident has essentially lost the will to live. In some cases, this phase can last several weeks or even months. If we were not watching the resident closely, we might think his or her symptoms were merely a sign of fatigue—especially if no one brings up the question of approaching readiness for death. In other cases, the change is obvious. If a resident's state has been dwindling over a longer period, it is not as noticeable as when a resident has a sudden decline.

At this point, we have to judge whether the person's current condition has been brought on by physical factors, such as side effects from medicine (for example, the loss of taste) or infections, or is emotional, such as a sudden sadness. Once we rule out these other possible causes, we can establish that the resident is approaching readiness to die, and we communicate that with transparency to the staff. When the staff understand this, they can begin to act accordingly.

It is very important that we yield to the natural process the resident is undergoing and that we do not pressure the person to live a life that he or she no longer wants, especially one supported by all sorts of medical instruments. The nightmare scenario is the elderly care home resident who suddenly wakes up in an intensive care unit at a hospital, hooked up to every imaginable device. A person in this situation has usually been denied the right to say goodbye and die naturally. You might call it a kind of destructive extension of life.

The resident's interest in getting out of bed diminishes during this final phase of life. Some people will sleep around 20 hours a day. They do not stay awake for a moment longer than they want to, and it becomes increasingly difficult to get them up and moving, even after they have slept.

> We can reach even the most apprehensive family members when we talk about death in a straightforward, normalizing way.

Communicating with the Relatives

Once we are sure that a resident is approaching death, we inform the relatives. We tell them what we have observed and explain that these changes do not mean the resident is going to die tomorrow, but that he or she is heading in that general direction—and that we believe the person does not want to live anymore. We tell them that their loved one is not in pain and that there nothing else wrong with the person, but that the disease has naturally run its course. Only rarely have the relatives concluded it themselves at this stage. They might have had a gut feeling about it, and, when we tell them, they respond, "Ah, so that's what it is." But the majority are surprised by the news.

For the most part, if we are honest and explain that this shift is part of the natural process, then it is a good, and even easy, conversation to initiate with the relatives. We can reach even the most apprehensive family members when we talk about death in a straightforward, normalizing way. Some might be shocked but will put up a façade of understanding and acceptance. Therefore, we typically call them and give them an update a couple of days after our initial conversation. We want

Life at Our Home

"There's no reason to panic. I'm calling you because we've noticed that Ingrid's condition is worsening, and I wondered if you have time to talk about it." The other end of the line went silent before Ingrid's son sighed. He asked if I meant "now." I said it didn't have to be, but that we wanted to explain what was happening to his mother and her needs during the next stage. Ingrid's son, who was a CEO in a big company and was abroad for work, preferred to meet as soon as possible. He quickly ordered a ticket home and arrived the next day. We sat down and talked with him face to face. Our forthrightness seemed very new to him. I clearly explained our recent observations of his mother: her decreased appetite, how we had tried to address it, how she no longer felt like going outside, and so on. I told him it was part of a completely natural process; that we would help her through it; that in a couple of weeks his mother would probably be bedridden; and that, at that point, we would likely begin to administer some medicine for her pain and uneasiness. There was far too much information for him to process at that first meeting, so I told him we would keep him updated as the weeks passed. He thanked us profusely before going out to his car. He also remarked on how he was used to intense meetings with his work, but never with such a high level of transparency.

to be completely sure they understand the consequences of what we spoke about earlier. After that, the nurse will continue to refer to it in every exchange with the relatives, whether it is a conversation or during their visits.

It is important not to try to spare the relatives by giving them false hopes during this phase. Not talking openly about impending death deprives dying individuals of what feels natural to them and deprives their relatives of the opportunity to prepare themselves. The residents and their families are forced to keep hanging on. Instead, we need to encourage relatives to follow the resident's natural transition. There is a reason why a resident has become ready for life to end and has chosen to withdraw. He or she has had enough and willingly submits to the natural process. Residents with dementia deserve the same end as patients at a hospice, where it is generally accepted that they are there to end their lives. I am not saying I think the residents should be moved from the care home to a hospice in their final days, but that there should be the same nursing principles and framework around residents at a care home as there are for people who are dying at a hospice.

Changes in the Person

During this phase, a resident's waste matter will reveal some of the changes occurring in the body. The person does not need to go to the bathroom very often because he or she no longer eats very much. At the same time, the resident recognizes it as a sign that his or her own body is shutting down. In other words, the bodily functions have an effect on the resident's own understanding of the situation. This is OK; the resident surrenders to it.

For the most part, the resident does not suffer in this phase. He or she has some mobility and still eats a little—whatever strikes their fancy. The internal organs are still functioning; the person has not reached that critical point at which everything breaks down. Rather, the process of weakening is gradual. How long it takes, or exactly what happens during this process, is determined by the person's age and type of dementia. But the process is completely normal.

The resident now seems to exist on a slightly elevated, "spiritual" level and does not want us to disturb the process he or she is undergoing. We see something in the person's gaze, as if he or she is already looking down on us from above. The resident acknowledges that we are there, but the person is somewhere else; after all, he or she knows better than we do, as this is the person's journey. I feel it is important to experience our residents during this beautiful phase. We do not work to include them in all sorts of activities that would tear them away from their current state. The message they send to us is loud and clear: "Let me be, but keep living around me." We make way for their process of dying. We welcome it and recognize it as it appears in each individual resident.

The resident in this stage deserves peace and quiet. Admittedly, allowing it can be difficult for those of us who care for the person, as we are inclined to keep engaging until we are absolutely certain we cannot and should not. The stage that I have described above is first noted after a longer period during which we have gone to great lengths to ensure the resident kept eating, drinking, and participating in the life of the home.

Determining whether or not a resident is approaching readiness for death is not a decision we make from one day to the next. It is gradual and ongoing, and we do not rule out the possibility of a sudden return. We have seen that happen as well. A person can suddenly revive after displaying the above-mentioned symptoms for an extended period. These sudden turnarounds are often short-lived and occur right before death. We allow space for this renewal, of course, without having too many expectations. The resident might suddenly regain skills not seen for a while, and this sudden state of activity can occur right up until his or her final bedrest. The resident may well have been bedridden, and then suddenly wake up and remember names, numbers, and all sorts of things. Usually, things quickly decline again, even if the resident both ate and drank during his or her brief comeback. It is difficult to pinpoint exactly when these kinds of upswings will occur, and yet it happens more often than not. Perhaps it is the last vestiges of the person's survival instinct.

The Norm:
Pressure Ulcers, Yogurt, and a Failure to Act

Why would we say that we want the best for our elders in decline and then barely react when they finally signal they are ready for life to end, and that they want to die? It may be just avoidance of something difficult, or it may be ignorance. For many, it can be a fear of deciding what the signals are telling them, based on their own intuition and professional judgment.

During the weakening phase, the usual task checklist becomes meaningless, so what needs to be done from one moment to the next may be unclear. In addition to that uncertainty, the relatives, watching from the sidelines, may naturally find it hard to accept that their loved one is dying. They have high hopes and insist, "There must be something you can do." Meanwhile, the nurse or staff member may not have the words or the communication skills to broach the subject and explain the simple truth that their father is ready for life to end. He has stopped eating and drinking because he would like to die. It was meant to happen. We have to listen to him now.

Instead, the staff frantically rush around, almost mechanically. It is as if they are thinking, "Where's an open mouth I can stuff some yogurt into?" "Where's the journal so I can record what I've given him?" In the meantime, they overlook the resident himself, who is trying to tell them he cannot handle any more. He does not want yogurt, or any other food for that matter. There is no consideration of what is right before their eyes. Are there any signs? Why isn't he participating in the singalong anymore? Could it be that the singing and the group no longer have anything to offer him? The staff barge in and out of his room, loudly talking over his head, trying to jostle him back to his old self. This reflects a too-common lack of humility toward the dying individual's journey. Instead of making noise, try opening up for sensing; enable peace and quiet.

When, after all strategies that usually work—group singing, a glass of juice, or jokes—do not trigger a smile or even a reaction, what happens then? Often, a staff member in a normal care home will turn away, perhaps coming up with a slightly offended rationalization: "When he says he can't be bothered to get out of bed, why should I bother him?" He stays bedridden for weeks. At least then, that "difficult" resident will not be a problem anymore when he says he longer feels like participating in all the fun activities at the care home. The staff can resort to reporting the basics: when his incontinence pad was changed, what side he was lying on, what he normally drinks, and so on. They can stick to the charts.

This is often how the sated phase unfolds at a care home, and also why—for the majority of care home residents—the final course of the disease is long and grueling. They may lie in bed for a very long time, being fed yogurt and other mushy food. The staff might order a pressure-relief mattress to prevent pressure ulcers, because there is no avoiding them in these kinds of drawn-out deaths. A toilet stool stands next to the bed along with a pile of incontinence pads. A bowl may sit in the windowsill so that it is convenient to wipe down the person once in a while, if he or she does not seem too tired.

At this stage, the resident's room is often transformed into a lackluster hospital room, with pads, tubs, trash cans, yogurt, and protein drinks on the sickbed table. It is a scene of undignified chaos. It begins to feel natural to the staff to leave residents at this stage bedridden and alone in their room for long periods at a time—that is, until they get pneumonia or festering pressure ulcers on their heels or tailbone. These latter lead to unbearable nerve pain because the wounds are often close to the bone due to extreme weight loss. The resident now becomes the nurse's responsibility, and the focus is the status of the wound and replacing the antiseptic dressings.

A whole day can be spent discussing new balms and lotions to put on the wound. "Procedure performed by nurse" states the care documentation.

So, the resident lies in a stuffy room, tucked under a warm duvet, wearing a pad filled with runny and acidic excrement as a result of the monotonous yogurt diet. As the weeks drag on, the person is treated increasingly like a living corpse. The dying resident is disconnected both from his or her own life and the decision to end it.

A drawn-out bedrest redirects the focus on the medical issues and away from whatever the resident might have wanted. Another aspect of these scenarios is that the staff in the care home manage to display a complete lack of honesty with the relatives. They do not communicate why various precautions have been taken. Perhaps the staff members do not actually understand it themselves, so the information somehow never gets passed on to the family. Instead, it only adds to the medical commotion around the person in the bed. The relatives often find themselves in a losing battle during this period, desperate to get their mother or father out of bed again. They keep asking, "Is my mom getting out of her room today?" or "Her hair is greasy; can she get it washed?" A problematic relationship develops between the care staff and the relatives about what is possible or not, now that their mother is lying voiceless in bed.

All things considered, the situation is far from what it should be: a peaceful, calm, and dignified death. No one questions it. The prevailing view—another misconception—is that it is normal for people at a nursing home to die this way.

Objection:
"We don't play God."

The argument that the care home would be "playing God" by allowing someone to die naturally contradicts the only dignified and ethical thing to do, which is to honor the needs of that dying individual. Usually, no one wants to help the person make the final decision. Afraid, the staff absolve themselves of responsibility and leave the person's final days of living and dying in the hands of an impersonal system. The resident is forced to eat until he or she cannot be fed any longer and simply stops opening his or her mouth. Meanwhile, the person's signals are overlooked by the staff.

I think we often forget that our most important task in these cases is to listen to the resident. When the person shows us he or she cannot continue, it does not work to create empty incentives for pushing on. Our duty is to take the job of listening seriously and act. Care personnel are trained to be conscientious and respectful of a resident's self-determination in every other situation. Perhaps the caregivers forget that there is something bigger at stake when the person is getting ready to die. This human being wants us to stop the endless striving for solutions and procedures. Nursing has unfortunately gotten less nuanced; we are seldom asked to look at the bigger picture, beyond keeping a person's body alive.

Ethical questions are always problematic, especially if our colleagues do not see the virtue in considering different sides of an issue: "Peter doesn't want to eat or drink; he is tired, doesn't smile very often, and seems withdrawn. What do you think is happening? Is there something he wants to tell us? What do the rest of you think is the right thing to do at this point?" If you ask these questions, some colleagues will engage with them with an open mind, always considering the issue from the resident's perspective. Other colleagues will suggest different ways to get food into Peter's body.

Ethics are an important part of our professional judgment, but it is easy to forget to observe that aspect of our professional judgment in the daily rush to complete tasks and care for people with different conditions and in different stages of life. Ethics demands that we weigh every option—we do not play God. We take responsibility as care partners to respect a resident's wish to die and to leap alongside him or her with loving conviction. We do so because we care deeply about the resident, even at his or her worst—and we understand that "worst" is not necessarily a bad outcome.

Summary

Dying is a part of everyone's life. People without dementia are often able to know when they are ready to die, either from advanced age or illness, or suddenly, as a result of a trauma. People with dementia often die very slowly, and we must watch them closely to pick up the signs that their dying process has begun. All of our efforts before then are toward helping them stay healthy and engaged with life, but when we acknowledge that they are in the weakening phase, it is important to step back and support the person as best we can up until the end.

———————•◆•———————

Questions for Reflection

1. How do the staff in your organization manage a resident's approaching death? Describe not only the physical care that is given but also the emotional responses of care partners and their communication with the family.

2. Do you agree with the approach described in this chapter, to "step back" from trying to encourage the person to eat when he or she is no longer interested in doing so? What signals have you noticed that tell you a person is ready to die?

3. Are there ideas presented in this chapter that could be used in your organization to bring about a more peaceful experience for residents who are approaching death?

PART THREE

The Final Phase

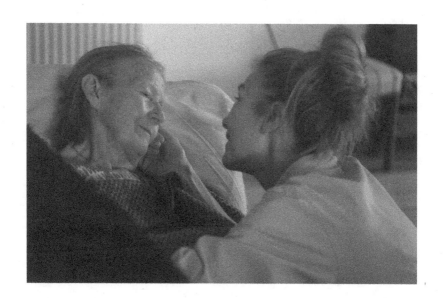

18

·◆·

Working with the Family

WE ARE IN THE FINAL stretch. As detailed in Chapter 17, we have observed a long period in which the resident has grown increasingly fatigued. He or she is apparently ready for life to end. But we have to be absolutely certain of that. Consequently, we discuss and reassess the state of this particular resident frequently. We ask ourselves and each other, "What can we tell from the signs? Is there any chance she might improve, that she will regain the will to live? Is it irreversible?" In the weeks leading up to this point, we have tried everything—offered more food, especially small cakes, candy, and other treats. We have tried taking the person for short trips around the garden and tried finding something that would catch her eye—anything that would cheer her up. If she does not respond to anything we do and does not want to come back to us, then it is our job as health professionals to listen to her.

Her expression has changed. She has become stony-faced and introverted. She rarely looks up to catch our eye. She is not interested in getting up in the morning. The shared activities do not seem to offer her anything, either. The resident does not necessarily appear sad; rather, she seems to be acknowledging to herself that she is slipping away. When we have reached a conclusion, based on our professional assessment of the situation, to let the resident lead us toward the end, she will typically withdraw even more. It is as though our acceptance allows the person to relinquish the last ties, as though she no longer needs to try. She does not want to eat or drink, and after a couple of days with barely any nourishment or fluids, she is at ease and quietly and calmly transitions to the next stage.

> *If we do not compassionately include the family members along the way, they end up worn out and distraught, not having slept for days, and their tension follows them into the dying resident's room.*

Supporting the Family

It will usually take a few weeks for a resident to die. We talk to the relatives and explain to them that we are now in the last phase of their loved one's disease. We also explain what we anticipate during the final days. We are very open with them about any clinical observations, so the family constantly feel clued in. For example, the nurse might say, "In a couple of days you might notice her getting more tired and sleeping longer. She will be bedridden and seem to be slipping farther and farther out of reach. Therefore, I recommend stopping by more frequently, so you can keep in close contact with her. That does not necessarily mean you have to stay by her side around the clock. Save your strength for the end. Go home and get some sleep; we will let you know when the time comes." When we speak honestly and candidly, the relatives become more accepting and less anxious about the situation. This is essentially to help the one who is dying. If we do not compassionately include the family members along the way, they end up worn out and distraught, not having slept for days, and their tension follows them into the dying resident's room.

Meanwhile, the staff continually prepare for any challenges that might arise, always keeping the relatives updated.

The relatives of a dying family member are often grieving for what they are about to lose. They might be feeling confused and inept, and consequently not be thinking clearly. As a result of the stressful situation they are facing, they will often have problems receiving information or will forget entirely what we have told them. Therefore, we may have to continually repeat the information we share with them—even if they seem perfectly alert. If we do not take care to communicate in this way, hours before the resident's death we might find ourselves facing a group of perplexed relatives, who feel both disappointed and caught unawares. It creates a difficult scene and an unhealthy power struggle, which should be avoided at all costs.

This is why I recommend always assigning one or two competent permanent employees the job of communicating with the family. These employees will take whatever time is needed to talk things over with the family. If too many people are involved in this communication, confusion or mixed messages can arise.

All of the staff need to be informed when a resident is nearing death. There is no point in agreeing on something with the relatives if everyone onsite is not informed. Something as rudimentary as agreeing that a resident no longer receives fluids needs to be understood by staff and relatives alike. The family needs to know exactly why we have decided to stop giving the resident anything to eat or drink. They need to know that we are not trying to kill their loved one. Rather, it is because during this weakening phase, the person no longer needs nourishment or fluids. He or she is going to die soon. For the same reason, we do not administer intravenous (IV) fluids. We need to ensure that the resident can pass away as easily as possible. Death becomes less painful and calmer, and there are fewer complications during the final hours, if we do not offer fluids of any kind. Mere drops of solution or juice can add several days—days filled with pain and discomfort for the dying.

Life at Our Home

The wife of one of our residents came for a visit. Her husband was in the final stages of his disease and had been asleep for a week. He was in a coma and unresponsive. He had been like that for a couple of days while his wife stopped by every day. She was grief-ridden, and although the prognosis was obvious, her husband's dying didn't seem to get through to her despite our attempts to communicate it.

On this day, she came into her husband's room with a bag of homemade rolls. The staff were touched by the gesture, impressed by her surplus energy at a time like this. It wasn't the first time she had brought homemade goods to our home. The wife went to her husband's side and said, "Look, dear, I brought you some of those rolls you love." The staff member in the room went to her and put her hands on the woman's shoulders and praised her for the rolls, but reminded her that her husband wasn't going to eat them now. "He is dying and we don't think he will wake up again. But listen, he can probably still smell them, and feels loved knowing you've made them for him and that you're here by his side." That episode was a turning point for her, ending her anxious denial. Instead, she took on the role of a wife who was experiencing the death of her husband and sharing his last moments.

The family's only task during the final period of a resident's life is to be close to their loved one. They should not be caregivers who have to make decisions about the body's dwindling functions, or about which medicine would be most effective for pain relief, and so on. They should not be sitting at the bedside on their own trying to figure out if death can be averted. The staff know it is not possible, and their certainty can actually be a source of strength to the family. This is why the nurse needs to make sure the family understands that direct care is the staff's responsibility and that the family should spend their time talking and being with the resident, gaining a deeper understanding of what is going to happen. They need to trust that the resident is in good hands, and should therefore also sense and see that it is.

The Norm:
Silence and Confusion in the Halls

All of us in the care sector need to remember that a loved one's death is not an everyday occurrence for most people. We have to treat the resident and his or her family with the utmost respect and kindness, and also provide clear and complete communication. Unfortunately, this is often not the norm in most nursing homes. Following is an account from a relative who described how painful it can be when health professionals and relatives talk past each other—when the staff has failed to gain the family's trust.

"Treatment level!" I had no idea what the nurse in charge at the care home was talking about. I thought we'd agreed on a treatment level at a meeting with her and the general practitioner a couple of months before, when we needed to decide whether or not we were going to resuscitate my mother in case of a heart attack.

So, late that Friday afternoon, I felt as if I were back to square one. Around 2:00, I decided to stick my head into the care home's main office to voice my concerns. My mother, who had Alzheimer's disease, had recently been suffering from a bladder infection. They had given her antibiotics, but she hadn't improved and hadn't eaten or drunk much. Even though they said they were charting her fluid balance, that afternoon I discovered she had hardly had anything to drink the whole day.

This concerned me, because I know how important it is to drink plenty of liquids after a bladder infection. At least that's what you hear. I must have looked like one big question mark, standing there in the doorway of the office. So, the nurse repeated in a loud voice, "I said, we need to talk about a treatment level!"

"But I thought we already did. I just want my mom to get some more fluids," I tried to explain. Then I suddenly realized, that wasn't what she meant. But she never *explained* what she actually meant. Instead, she almost appeared angry. So, I asked her to get hold of a doctor; otherwise, I was sure my mom was going to die of thirst that weekend. When I insisted that my mom be put on IV fluids, she reluctantly called my mother's doctor. The doctor had already gone home for the weekend.

I moistened my mother's lips with a damp sponge. I didn't dare give her a sip from the sippy cup because she'd started showing signs of "dysphagia"—one term among many that we had to learn. I couldn't understand why they didn't just hydrate my mother. I complained to one of my mom's regular caregivers. From what I understood, my mother was just going to lie there and die of hunger and thirst. The caregiver tried to comfort me, explaining that the reason they didn't give her an IV was because my mother could "drown." *Drown!* No one ever had said anything about that—not until then, not that I understood what it meant.

After the weekend, the care home staff contacted my mother's doctor, who authorized the use of an IV. The doctor didn't seem to think there was any danger of the IV drowning my mom. She never fully recovered from that weekend. She kept getting weaker. The additional fluids from the IV only slightly helped, and it gradually got harder for her to swallow the blended food or protein drinks.

Some time later the doctor arrived, her heels hammering down the hall. She pulled up a little stool and sat down in front of us, still wearing her winter jacket, flanked by a nurse and another employee, and told me, in a very no-nonsense manner: "One of my patients is in critical condition, so I don't have much time. Your mom isn't improving, even after the fluids, so I don't think there's any point in continuing. It's time to accept your mother is now terminal."

That was the bottom line, bluntly communicated by a busy doctor: Your mother is going to die. The doctor quickly rushed off with the rest of the staff. We were left to our own devices, there in the reception hall for dementia patients, which looked more like the furniture section of the local thrift store. Slightly dazed, I looked around and asked myself when they were going to stop making these places look like something out of an old stuffy TV series. We were in shock. My mother's sudden pending death from Alzheimer's caught us off guard, although we'd always known it was coming. The fact that it was coming now was hard to swallow.

We went back to my mother's room. She looked so tiny and fragile in her bed. You could tell she sensed our presence. After everything, I still had this awful feeling my mother was going to die more from hunger and thirst than anything else. And there was nothing we could do. I sat down and kept moistening her lips with a damp sponge.

It can be a confusing time for both the staff and the relatives. Often, the confusion is caused by nurses forgetting to inform not only the relatives, but also the rest of the employees, about what is happening and about the various agreements concerning the resident's faltering health. It leads to chaos and inconsistent care, as in the account above, when the doctor chose a strategy that was lifesaving, but was different from the care strategy devised by the nursing home staff.

The direct care staff may understand that one of the bedridden residents is dying. But they may not have been informed about what kind of treatment the person needs at this time. "What the heck are we supposed to do? Should we give him something to drink, sit him up, change his pad?" It can quickly become messy and chaotic. If the staff do not address the problem and have not been given specific guidelines and plans, and no one has discussed these with the relatives, then the family can end up discovering by themselves that their loved one is on the brink of death. This is where they meet that clunky response: "We need to talk about a treatment level." It can be a weird and anxious conversation, in which the staff members do not take any responsibility to tell the family what they should do. The family is left in an awkward position, asking themselves what they should do, what they have to do, what the nursing home expects, and what the dying one expects. They think, "Should we sit and hold my mother's hand 24 hours a day from now on?"

There is seldom a role model among the staff who reaches out to the relatives, even if death and the care of the dying are fundamental to the career the staff members have chosen. It is a situation the personnel at care homes constantly encounter. It should by now be a well-coordinated, familiar exercise.

Instead, we see the staff frantically rushing in and out of the room. The relatives are left on their own, "pacified" with a bell they can ring if they need help—despite the fact that they are in mourning and may be incapable of deciding what they might need help for.

Objections:
"But we informed the relatives . . ."

No one would consciously choose to deny a person the right to pass away with their well-informed and fully assured family by their side. Nevertheless, deaths in many nursing homes are chaotic and traumatic for all involved. I can only assume the staff believe they have done their best. If the staff overlook, or are not trained to recognize, a resident's signs of being ready for life to end, then vital conversations never come up at the staff meetings. We need to have conversations about ethics, in which we delve into the pros and cons of the situation, and, as a group, identify and plan for the upcoming course of the disease. Then, as staff go about their work in the home, everyone is working with the same understanding and expectations.

Without that common ground among the staff, it can become difficult to maintain clear and consistent communication with the relatives. The reality is that the parameters for care probably exist somewhere in most nursing homes, listed in bullet point form. For example, the staff think that the relatives have been informed because they see a note from the nurse in the journal stating: "Talked to the daughter, Hanne, yesterday. Informed her about the treatment level." But that documentation is inadequate for the situation. Staff might truly believe the relatives are fully up to date. But confronting the family's grief and their existential questions means that the ethics and morality involved in the end of a life cannot just be checked off a list. We must never assume that the relatives are on the same page as we are, especially if we communicate using our own clinical terminology, which, when it comes down to it, is often there just for legal reasons to protect the staff. If ever anyone contends that the staff did something wrong, our backs are covered. However, our backs are not really covered if the families we abandon are in pieces and in crisis from having been dragged through an environment which, frankly speaking, reduces the dying resident to a car at the mechanic shop.

My advice: Forget your back and turn around. Be willing to have those hard conversations, both at the staff meetings and with the relatives. Get to the heart of the expectations and hopes for the resident, so that he or she can die in peace and comfort, in the company of loved ones at their best.

Summary

It is difficult knowing someone we love is going to die. Death is not a normal part of everyday life for most families, and as health professionals we need to keep this in mind. We also need to remember that our handling of this phase is critical—not only for the one dying, but also for the relatives.

---◆◆◆---

Questions for Reflection

1. In this chapter, the author argues against the idea of treating dying as a medical problem to solve. What are your feelings and thoughts about her approach?

2. How does your organization's approach to families differ from that of Dagmarsminde? What are some similarities?

3. Is the dying process of a resident "a well-coordinated, familiar exercise" at your care home, or is there a sense of crisis or confusion among staff, families, or residents when someone is dying? Describe your ideal of this process, as it might look in your care home.

19

---•◆•---

The Dying Process

WE ARE APPROACHING THE END of the road. Of late, the resident has shown us where he or she wants to go—the end of life. Our duty is to ensure that the person's journey is as comfortable and easy as possible. At Dagmarsminde, we have a specific framework for the final period. Our ethos is built on our experience, our professional knowledge, and ethical considerations. As discussed in Chapter 18, when everyone is aware of the course of events, we avoid accidents and misunderstandings. Making sure that all staff members understand their tasks and exactly when each will be needed gives the dying resident and his or her family peace of mind and reassurance. In this chapter, I describe our approach to the final days, hours, and minutes leading up to the resident's last breath.

It is important to keep in mind that customs and laws regarding care for the dying and recently deceased will vary widely throughout the world. What follows is a description of how we work at Dagmarsminde.

Days Until Life's End

We begin with the practical matters. First, our general practitioner confirms that the condition of the individual in question is *terminal*. He fills out the Dying Declaration. Among other things, this document states that there are no longer grounds for treatment, as the patient is not expected to live for much longer. The declaration is also recognized as a release to obtain any medication that might be needed at the end. The medicine is expensive, but in Denmark at least, with a doctor's declaration, it is free of cost for the resident's family.

Action Plan

The Dying Declaration becomes a kind of harbinger—an initiation of our treatment and care. We set up a plan of action in our journal system to indicate we are heading into a terminal situation. One of the entries in our plan is called "worsening of the general condition during the terminal phase"; this is where we note down everything about the dying individual.

At this point, when the resident only has a few days left to live, he or she is bedridden, and specific staff members are assigned to care for the resident and family. We make sure that whoever is appointed can focus entirely on the resident and his or her family.

It is crucial that the staff member who is in charge of the direct care is a health professional with a solid background. One trained nurse from our regular staff is placed in charge for all shifts. She makes all executive decisions and delegates duties to the rest of the staff. It is also primarily the nurse who stays in the resident's room throughout.

We usually call in extra staff to cover the duties that would otherwise be covered by the nurse during this period. We set aside specific funds for additional staffing costs that occur during the terminal cases. This is not a common practice at most care homes, but we prioritize it because we think it is important for the final care, which can often be complicated, to be provided by someone with extensive nursing experience.

The nurse has the knowledge to administer medicine and perceive its effect—maintaining a balanced and suitable level of drugs—and also has the most experience interpreting the different gestures and signs of someone who is dying. Although she enlists the help of other staff, she is the one who handles and stays the course until the end. She is also the one who contacts the family to make sure their wishes are heard.

Medication and Assistive Devices

The doctor prescribes medications that the resident needs in connection with complications related to bedrest and dying. These are primarily sedatives, pain relievers, and diuretics, administered either as a suppository or through an injection. We do not call the family and tell them, "We've just requested drugs for the terminal phase." That is too clinical. Instead, we explain, in plain words, when and why certain drugs will be necessary.

It is important to order the medication in good time so that it is available in case the need arises suddenly. We make sure that our general practitioner requests it, so that we do not have to make an emergency request to a doctor with no previous knowledge of the resident.

We also order and request certain assistive devices, which we know from experience are necessary; these include a hospital bed, because residents sleep heavily during their final hours, and a pressure-relieving mattress to avoid pressure ulcers. Everything needs to be ready before the time comes. If the mattress is not ordered in time, the dying resident would have to be transferred in their final hours—which disturbs the transition to death.

In much the same manner, we make sure all the paraphernalia is ready: needles, tubs, washcloths, mouth swabs, and so on. When we have everything on hand, we redirect our attention to our main focus: the person and his or her family. As with most aspects of our care at Dagmarsminde, when all the basic elements are in order, we are free to go more deeply into our work.

Observation

At this point, our greatest concern is keeping the resident out of the hospital. One of our core values is that residents should die at home. We set up a tiny "invisible workspace" in the room, so we do not have to go in and out all the time. This space consists of a little shelf inside a closet; we hook up a lamp and arrange the various supplies needed, so they are not spread around the room. Needles and other paraphernalia lined up along the bedside would make the room feel institutional and alienating to the resident.

This period after the Dying Declaration is signed usually lasts around a week. In the first couple of days, it is okay to check in on the person from time to time while he or she is calmly sleeping. But during the last few days, someone stays in the room with the relatives around the clock. This is another reason why we create our little space, where we can sit with a computer and document, for example, the medicine being administered, which requires constant charting. Dosage of medication and its effects have to be recorded immediately, because we usually administer it at frequent intervals.

Beyond medication, we observe the resident constantly for any signs of unease, pain, or breathing problems. We are very firm about any direct care being done by the staff. This includes the meticulous oral hygiene, personal care, change of clothes, incontinence pads, sheets, and so on. The family is not there to provide care, not even wiping away saliva, during their last hours with their loved one.

However, some relatives may want to provide some sort of care. In those cases, we suggest some of the nicer things they can do for the dying resident. These might include combing the person's hair, applying lip balm, or moisturizing their hands with some nice cream. We only present these options if the relatives really want to provide care. We make absolutely no demands. The family should never have to handle the difficult direct care tasks. They are present as relatives and should be allowed to embrace a more spiritual, familial role.

Being there to support and guide the family is partly also a way of preserving the resident's integrity. One woman had a hard time accepting that her mother was dying and had found peace; we saw her trying to pry her mother's eyes open and shouting, "Mom, are you there?" We are there to ensure that the dying resident's final existence is calm and peaceful in every way, and everyone is clear about what is happening. We talk to the family members about the signs and symptoms we observe. We do this so they do not suddenly feel as if we are encroaching upon the dying resident when we reposition him or administer medication.

When we observe signs that the resident is in pain—furrows on the person's brow or a worried expression—we need to respond. The resident is often in a coma for the last few days of life, and then we only have facial expressions, twitches in the hands or legs, or trembling to show us he or she is in pain. The resident might also let out a sound. We do not know if this is caused by pain, but we believe so, and therefore we respond accordingly. The resident suffers from being bedridden. Even slight adjustments of position can cause him or her great discomfort. We would rather administer some sort of pain relief than have the resident experience more pain. Our goal is to keep the person's relief from pain constant. Here are some signs a dying person is in pain:

- Sighing and moaning
- Angry facial expressions
- Narrowed eyes
- Furrowed brow
- Clenched fists
- Tense muscles
- Twitching limbs and the face
- Twitching eyelids
- Hyperextended arms and legs
- Clenched jaw
- Grinding teeth
- Sudden skin color changes, for example, on the face

A select few residents are awake until the very last moment, but most remain in a coma, partly because they are medicated. As I discussed earlier, we are normally not in favor of medicating our residents, but because of their dementia, they often get very uneasy, anxious, or even outright tormented right before they die. This may be a result of their underlying illness making it difficult for them to understand the situation in moments of awareness. People with dementia are also more likely to become delirious than other older people, especially when they have not had anything to eat or drink for a couple of days. They can hallucinate and suffer from paranoid delusions.

With only a very few days left to live, the resident now needs calm and rest. We need to allay their angst and any pain. At this point, our regular care treatment is not enough to relieve the resident from discomfort because they are asleep and unreachable, so we often have to medicate them.

We know that when the resident stops waking up when we try to move him or her, then the person is close to passing away. He or she has no energy left and cannot see, take part in life, or express much of anything. As the person's expression gets harder and harder to read, even a tiny furrow or twitch around the eye is essential for us to pick up on, as it might be a cue for us to reposition an arm, regulate the temperature in the room, or administer more pain relief. The family members do not always catch these signs, which is another reason why we always have a staff member in the room. We have to react quickly, before any pain progresses.

Throughout the dying process, we make sure to communicate our observations to the family: "Your mother's brow is starting to furrow—she might be experiencing pain of some sort, so it is time for us to administer some pain-relief drugs to minimize her suffering." We are careful not to sound didactic or condescending. We keep the conversation open and honest when giving information and responding to any doubts or questions raised by the family.

A resident's breathing may become labored and noisy if they have fluid in their lungs; this is not unusual for people who are dying. At Dagmarsminde, we never allow these kinds of sounds to persist. We cannot be absolutely certain they indicate discomfort, but we also do not want the person to lie there sighing and possibly in pain. Therefore, we try to adjust the position of the resident in bed, or we will administer medication if that does not work. Our goal is to help the resident sleep and rest as much as possible, and medication is essential during these final days. It is also partly for the family's sake that we try to mitigate their loved one's increasingly intense respiration. The resident may no longer actually sense this kind of discomfort, but the sound can make the family apprehensive and distraught at a time when the resident needs them most.

It is common for residents to have bad breath in their final days. This is caused by fasting and the so-called ketone bodies released by the body during the process. The smell is slightly sweet or like rubbing alcohol, and the more loudly and deeply they breathe, the stronger the smell is.

As you can see, we try to ease the pressure from the dying and give the family a calm, peaceful last few days with their loved one, enabling them to say goodbye as they wish.

Life at Our Home

Another nurse and I were in the room of a resident on the last day before she died. There were three family members present. The atmosphere in the room was calm, with quiet music in the background and warm, quiet conversations. It was time for us to reposition their mother in her bed. She was fast asleep, and her breathing was calm and steady. But as soon as we turned her on her side, she suddenly got sick. She grew pale, sweaty, and after letting out a high-pitched sound, she stopped breathing for a couple of minutes. The family were startled and rushed to her side in panic. "Is she dying now?" As the resident's pulse gradually stabilized, we helped the family members calm down. Ever since that experience, whenever we are repositioning a resident in the dying phase, we make sure to medicate the person beforehand, regardless of how at ease they may seem before the move. We tell the family that the resident may physically react to the repositioning and that it may be uncomfortable for them to witness. We ask if they would prefer to be present or wait outside for a moment. If they choose the latter, we assure them that if they are close by, they will immediately be called back if the resident succumbs while being moved.

I previously noted the importance of preparing the room for the comfort of the dying individual and their family. That is why we have a section in our core values called "Light, sound, and creating a peaceful environment for the dying." We believe it is important to consider the space where the resident will die. It needs to feel normal. For the resident, that space is unquestionably their room in the care home, their own private space. The only change we make is moving the bed away from the wall, so that the staff and the family can stand or sit on both sides. This might make it look like a hospital bed, but it is better than having to move the bed back and forth whenever we need to get close to the resident. If the resident does not have any chairs in his or her room, we fetch some comfortable ones from the shared living space, so the family can easily stay for long stretches of time. We also have some lounge beds, which we set up in the room, in case the relatives themselves need to rest.

> *A normal, clean, and neat environment gives peace of mind to everyone in the room.*

The room needs to be tidy, neat, and welcoming, exactly as it always is. Our aesthetic values do not change just because a resident is dying. We are always tidying, so there are no piles or messes anywhere. We are not at a hospital, and the situation was anticipated and is perfectly normal. A normal, clean, and neat environment gives peace of mind to everyone in the room. In addition, unless the family would prefer otherwise, we use a diffuser to scent the room with a calming essential oil such as rose or lavender, sometimes mixed with a drop of Douglas fir. At times, we play calming music. We pay attention to and regulate it to suit the moment.

Maintaining the Rhythm of Life

I would briefly like to return to the subject of a resident's circadian rhythm. Out of respect for the dying person, it is important that we continue the same routines to which he or she is accustomed. This means that we draw the curtains at night and open them the next morning. The curtain becomes symbolic of the subtle transitions the resident is going through. The person needs to sense the daylight and the fresh breeze coming through the window, although it is only slightly ajar. In the evening, we turn on a few small cozy lamps in the room, or even light candles if it seems fitting—remembering not to go overboard, as we do not want the room to look eerie.

Our voices remain unchanged. There is no point in whispering or mysteriously tiptoeing around as though danger is right around the corner. We might even directly advise the relatives to speak in a normal tone of voice: "It's important, because your father might still be able to sense and hear you. He might not understand what you're saying, but your voice adds to the ambiance in the room. So, if you're sitting here talking and laughing about something, please don't stop—especially if it's concerning experiences you've had with your father. Or feel free to talk about happenings within the wider family; let it sound like a family reunion around the bed. It's nice." Lightening the mood is comforting to the resident, as well as to the family and staff. It is helpful to keep in mind, though, that the dying resident's hearing may be impaired. In that case, relatives have to remember to get up close when they want their loved one to hear them.

Sometimes it is difficult to keep the mood light and normal in a room with a dying relative. There are naturally times when people will grieve and cry, and of course we allow time and emotional space for that as well.

Forbearance

The nursing staff need to show empathy and sympathy at all times—even if the relatives sometimes interrupt our professional deliberations concerning the resident's complications. The staff need to accept it as part of the process and not allow themselves to characterize the relatives as irritating; usually, they are simply trying to cope under the enormous mental strain.

At our staff meetings, we talk about how the situation requires a certain amount of forbearance. The relatives come to us with countless questions, from a point of either sorrow or fear, and then we have to respond in more depth than we might otherwise. But we do not want these conversations to turn into an outright argument in the middle of our living spaces. Understandably, when someone is afraid, he or she will need a little extra reassurance that everything is in order. We have had relatives who lost family members in the past and, because of that, have felt abandoned. Consequently, they are more sensitive about the situation. They are terrified of being abandoned again, nervous about whether or not they can trust us and whether we will do what we promise.

At the same time, the staff must remember what their role is. The personnel are not a part of the family, so we keep a distance at farewells, we do not sit down among them as they reminisce; rather, we keep to ourselves. We allow the family to be alone together, but we stay nearby and at their disposal. We are constantly on call.

We have to attend to the dying individual's needs, but sometimes we discover the family themselves need a break. If we can see that the resident is not just about to die, we often recommend that the relatives go home and rest. We tell them we do not think anything is going to happen right away, and that we will call them if anything changes. In that case, they should be prepared to come quickly. If the family wants to stay, then we suggest they take a short walk outside and get some fresh air. No relative can stand being needed on a constant basis. The family should not sleep in the resident's room for days either; it simply is not good for them. It is only on the last night or, at most, the last two nights that they stay and sleep next to the dying resident.

We do not use volunteer night nurses at Dagmarsminde. We are always there ourselves. I am not actually a fan of night nurses when it comes to watching over people with dementia. Caring for our residents is complicated and constant; it is a job that requires a trained health professional.

We sometimes have to remind the relatives of the resident's need for some "alone time." The dying individual needs human contact and touch, but not around the clock. They may exert themselves when the family is around all the time; it can get very intense for them. We might step in and counsel the family from time to time. For example, if they keep stroking the resident's arm, we suggest they take a little break, because it might be uncomfortable for the resident to be touched in the same place repeatedly—perhaps they should try the other arm or softly press down on different areas of the body.

Throughout the dying process, whenever the relatives are present, the staff members need to remember to offer them some food and something to drink. Our staff will enter the room with a tray and offer a little nourishment from time to time, making sure it is substantial—not just a couple of dry crackers, but real food. They need the energy, as well as the care. It can be enormously strenuous for relatives to sit by a resident's bedside for hours upon end.

Toward the end of the dying process, we make sure the family is fully aware that their loved one may take their last dying breath without them by their side. It happens sometimes, and I think it happens partly because the dying resident was finally left in peace to die. He or she no longer feels it necessary to hang on for the family's sake. Having a lot of activity with people around can also prolong the process of dying. Once in a while, the residents need a little help to die peacefully in their sleep. From time to time, we simply have to test it out. If the resident is showing signs of exhaustion from the family's presence, we might say: "Some peace and quiet now may help your mother pass away." If death occurs while the family is gone, then we help them see that maybe it was for the best.

Care for the Body During the Dying Process

Positioning and caring for the body of the dying resident is crucial during their final days. The dying individual needs to be placed in the bed as if it were a nest—a nest for dying. We tuck the covers and pillows around him or her, and we also wrap a long body pillow, usually used in pregnancy, around the resident. The person's entire body is cushioned and unable to fall or roll out. The pillow over him or her provides a feeling of safety and security.

It is important to remember to check the person's temperature periodically. If the resident is covered by a duvet, then give the duvet an occasional shake and turn it over. The resident often gets very hot as a result of the medication, so sometimes only a sheet is needed.

The resident's appearance should be maintained at all times. We dab the resident's body with soft warm washcloths, wash and comb the hair, and apply moisturizer to the skin. We perform these tasks step by step, making sure the resident's body is covered with a cloth throughout, and explaining to the person what we are doing along the way.

We might bring along an object, perhaps something that smells familiar, from the person's spouse or other member of the family. When one of our male residents was dying, we placed his wife's scarf next to him in his bed, and he suddenly reacted to her scent. This practice is common among those who work with premature babies; the caregivers place a piece of the mother's clothes or an object next to the infant. This also works well with the dying, and it is a comfort to the family. Some family members even feel like lying down next to their loved one to be as close as possible; they are more than welcome to do this—children or grandchildren especially may lie down beside the dying resident for a little while.

Final Preparations

The family needs to decide which clothes their loved one should wear after they have passed away. But we always err on the side of caution before asking. If we talk about this too soon, it might seem slightly obtuse. It can sound harsh to ask, "Have you considered what clothes your mother will be wearing in her coffin?" It is often best to talk to the family about the clothes right after the death. But if the family members have seemed overwhelmed, and have had to go home to rest or get their bearings, then we make sure to ask before. Sometimes they are in no position to pick out an outfit. In those cases, we might offer to help select those pieces the person always looked good in or find that cardigan he or she loved so much.

Some dying residents seem to struggle, as if they are afraid to let go. For others, it is easier, and they face it stoically. Personally, I think whether or not the death itself is easy has a lot to do with the resident's notion of death during their lives. If someone has always been very anxious about it, then it is harder for them to let go. It is never easy to prepare a resident who has dementia for death. You never really get to talk to them about it in advance, or they do not understand it when you try. The relatives need to understand that it is alright for them to tell their dying spouse, mother, or father to close their eyes and find peace. From time to time, we have to prompt them, if they cannot get themselves to say it. But for others, it comes naturally.

The Occurrence of Death

We can often tell that death is occurring by changes that appear in the resident's face. People often say the face looks "pointy." The external features of the face that stick out, especially the nose, suddenly become lighter as the blood drains.

The person's breathing also changes. It might stop and start again after several minutes. When it restarts, it can sound like a very deep sigh. Then it may stop again, and the relatives sit and wait—often anxiously—for the next breath.

After this, the breathing becomes shallow, as if the dying person cannot get enough air, and their breathing is restricted to the top of the throat. It sounds as though the person is quietly panting. Sometimes, though, they seem to be gasping for air—often because they haven't been sufficiently medicated—and they end up with panicky, "choked" breaths. Soon afterward, the face grows paler as the blood drains from the smaller veins in the skin. The resident's heart stops pumping blood around the body, and we can see a "wax doll" appearance as the muscles slacken, causing the wrinkles to smooth away and making the person look younger.

One of the assigned staff members is almost always there by the resident's bedside when death occurs. We support the relatives throughout unless they would rather be alone at that moment.

Immediately after the resident has passed away, we keep to the back of the room but continue looking after the relatives, observing how they respond individually and as a group. In general, we confirm the death out loud after the person has drawn his or her last breath, and then we open the window. We do not need to explain why. The relatives understand it as a symbolic gesture in our culture—we open the window for the soul to pass through.

Afterward, there is generally a feeling of disbandment. The family compose themselves and gradually get up and walk around a little—which is also when we help them find their way out of the room. If we do not help in this way, they will often feel compelled to stay. After half an hour, we suggest they take a walk or sit down in our shared living space for a cup of coffee, so that we can tend to their loved one. When they come back a little later, we have washed the resident, dressed him or her in their nicest clothes, and fixed their hair. If the hair is greasy, we wash it with dry shampoo. We do our utmost to ensure the resident is presentable. We remove the used linens and make the bed afresh. Everything needs to be dry and clean. We cover the deceased with a white sheet up to the chest and let it fall down over the edge of the bed, so it looks neat and elegant. We also place some flowers in the person's hands, which we fold over the chest.

Leading up to and right before the moment of death, we make sure to close the resident's eyes. It has to be done right before death occurs, or shortly after the final breath. The mouth is more difficult to adjust. We can close it if the family leaves relatively quickly, because then we can place something under the chin to keep the mouth closed; in the past, attendants tied the head of the person who had just died to keep everything in place, but that is not a common practice anymore because it leaves a mark on the skin. We raise the head of the bed slightly so that the resident's head tilts forward, closing the jaw; sometimes we place a pillow under the chin so that the mouth stays closed. If the resident has died on their side, then we let him or her remain in that position, if the family agree. There is no rule saying people have to die lying on their back.

We clean the room and light some candles, and then the family members come back inside to say goodbye. At this point, we have already outlined a plan for the family, so they know what kind of practical matters need taking care of. We call the undertaker because the family often prefer to leave that to us. Then the relatives go back home, and the resident remains in their room until the next day, when we hold a wake.

The Norm:
Alone in the Room with the Dying

Death often seems to sneak up unexpectedly on the staff of many care homes. The final weakening phase plays out before anyone realizes what is happening, and no one informs the relatives about what is up ahead. Likewise, there is seldom a health professional overseeing the process. This is because only rarely does a nursing home assign a staff member with the appropriate qualifications to care exclusively for the resident and his or her family during the final period. Many fail to acknowledge that attending to a person in the process of dying is a job that requires years of professional knowledge and experience.

Therefore, the events leading up to death are often frantic and chaotic. The course of the death reflects this. The dying individual is left to suffer pain, discomfort, and angst. It is undignified and without respect.

The quality of care at a given home varies depending on whoever is on duty. In a typical scenario, once it has suddenly become clear that a resident is dying, the person's private space is transformed into a hospital room, bursting at the seams with clinical instruments: toilet stools, lifts, incontinence pads, and nursing paraphernalia left lying around. The air is increasingly stuffy and filled with unpleasant odors. Once in a while, a staff member might step inside to handle the direct care with efficient, routine-driven movements, speaking in a loud voice without consideration for the resident who needs a pad change or needs to be repositioned, only to slip out again, calling over her shoulder, "Just give me a call if . . . ," her words echoing down the hall.

When should the family stop by? Should they have to make that decision on their own? The family needs a staff member making regular visits to the room, and at times, for them to stay. They need someone who can oversee the situation and be ready at all times to help. Instead, the personnel make sporadic visits. Often the staff will only take a quick peek inside the door and bark out a few contrived condolences to the relatives: "Stay close to her and keep talking to her. She feels your presence." Then, *voilà*, they're off again, having checked off the task of communicating with the relatives.

Too many families are left with the responsibility of figuring out what if anything to do, while feeling vulnerable and incapable of handling the situation. It is not uncommon for them to experience an intense trauma of their own, as they hear the dying resident loudly expressing his or her pain or fear. The relatives seldom question the way things unfold. Unfortunately, they may assume that this is the way people die these days. They believe the staff have a handle on things. However, for a variety of reasons, the staff member runs away from the very thing they were once taught to consider a virtue—helping people at their most vulnerable.

As I have stated previously, care homes need more trained nurses. The few who are hired are usually not allotted enough hours in their schedule to stay near the dying person, or to take a leading role in improving the care of the dying by discussing and collaborating across disciplines with the rest of the care staff in order to raise the quality of the care to a higher and more dynamic level. Instead, the nurse is constantly on the run, solving problems in several different places at once. Other staff can fill in or help, but they are neither trained nor have time to care for the dying.

Objection:
"We can't be at your father's
side the whole time."

Neither the politicians nor the individual care homes address
the issue of capacity for terminal cases, despite death being
a fundamental and natural part of working at a care home.
Is it too much to demand that our healthcare system ensure
that dying residents and their families are assisted by a health
professional when the time comes? Can't the healthcare system
demand that the staff enable it, and that the care home directors ensure it happens? As it stands now, dying residents in
care homes are low on the priority list.

When we hear about serious illnesses such as cancer or
heart disease, most would agree that these patients deserve
to die with dignity. It is also assumed that they will pass their
final days attended by health professionals at a well-equipped
hospice, surrounded by caregivers who are trained to care
for their physical and spiritual needs. What is the difference
between someone with dementia and someone dying of cancer?
I hear countless stories from relatives about terrible experiences surrounding the deaths of their loved ones. Why do these
traumatic deaths happen so often?

Perhaps it is because the staff feel overworked already or
do not understand the capabilities they have for caring for these
people. Perhaps leadership has told them they do not have the
"resources" to allow staff to take on more responsibility.

But set aside the resources jargon for a moment. Think
about what you really wish for your residents. No matter what
the constraints are in your organization, can you be there for
these people, a little more than you are now?

Summary

The topic of death is a major part of nursing and social science
studies. It takes up a lot of space in the syllabus and in our con-
science, yet more often than not, health professionals are not

actually involved in the direct care of the person with dementia who is dying, and in supporting his or her relatives. The family members are on their own, and many people with dementia who are dying receive medication too late, among other things, because the care staff are too occupied to call a nurse to administer the pain relievers or calming medications.

Caring for a dying human being is an enormous task, and we need to raise the bar if we wish to provide a more peaceful end. This involves careful planning once it is clear the resident is beginning to die. It requires clear and consistent communication among all staff as well as with the relatives, and close focus on the evolving needs of the person who is dying.

———— • ◆ • ————

Questions for Reflection

1. What, for you, is the biggest challenge with working with people who are dying, especially those with dementia? How can you work with that challenge?

2. Toward the end of this chapter, the author asks, "No matter what the constraints are in your organization, can you be there for these people, a little more than you are now?" Respond to that question yourself; include ways, large and small, in which you might be able to provide better care for residents who are dying than your organization typically does.

3. Everything the author describes in this chapter is legal and acceptable in Danish culture. In what ways do these practices differ from your culture, either for national or religious reasons?

20

The Wake

I ATTENDED A RESIDENT MEETING once at a large county care home, where both residents and their relatives were present. Everyone was crowded onto benches, while coffee, tea, and bowls of colorful chocolates were set out on tables. The care home's leaders had just finished presenting a customer satisfaction survey completed by the residents, which the directors summed up as "above average." When they were done showing various numbers and graphs, they asked the audience in the room if they had any questions.

One woman, a resident with a freshly cut bob, raised her hand. "I would like to know why no one ever says anything when one of us dies. Time and again, the residents vanish into thin air. I also wonder why the flag is flown at half-mast when the royals die, but not for us. It's a little unsettling, because sometimes I wonder what will happen when I die. Will anyone know I'm gone?" In a slightly patronizing tone, the director asked, "I'm sorry, what flagpole are we talking about . . .?"

The woman replied that it was the one she could see from her window. There were whispers across the tables, and people concluded she must have been talking about the flagpole over by the local Boy Scouts building. The care home did not have a flagpole. The director promised the resident that he would look into the possibility of purchasing a flagpole. Meanwhile, the woman never got an answer for why no one ever said anything when a resident passed away. The staff never mentioned it, and no one ever brought it up again (and that care home still does not have a flagpole).

The resident's question was actually highly relevant. Why would a care home make the subject of death taboo among the residents by not explaining the sudden disappearance of one of their neighbors? Perhaps the staff feel that it is not good for the residents to hear about death. However, this seems like a misplaced concern, as if death is something that needs to be swept under the carpet. Perhaps they assume that, since the residents are all fairly close to death, they probably do not want to hear about it. So they let the person die and then carry the coffin out the backdoor, so no one sees.

At Dagmarsminde, we always hold a wake after someone has died. It is a proud and respectful way of saying goodbye. And even though their passing is sad, it is also a kind of release. We honor the resident's life—the significance of that human life. And we make room for new life. Loss and hope are joined together, and the wake is symbolic of the eternal link between life and death. For us, as staff, watching as the casket is closed gives us a sense of wholeness.

Our residents are always informed when a fellow resident has died, and they join us at the wake. They all have had a connection to the resident. Regardless of whether they remember or not, the deceased was a companion and part of our little community. There is nothing strange about it for the remaining residents. On the contrary, they see it as a natural part of life. They know that people do not live forever, and they have attended many funerals throughout their long lives. They know what it means to lose someone, and they know the importance of respecting the person who no longer walks among us. The residents are often deeply affected and cry, but we comfort them, and they comfort each other.

The family decides what song we will sing. We make sure the undertaker performs the service at an appropriate time, enabling us all to participate. For the most part, it happens in the afternoon in our shared living space.

The coffin, already closed, is rolled out from the person's bedroom. We do not give a long speech, but merely say a few words about the resident. Then we sing, and afterwards have a toast with a little glass of port or non-alcoholic wine. The person has lived a long life, from crib to bed to coffin, and we were a part of it. It signifies the cycle of life.

Sometimes the resident's family bring flowers, and all the residents receive one, which they place on the coffin one after another. Then the coffin is placed into the hearse. Those residents who would like to walk behind the coffin as the undertaker heads up the driveway do so, and we stand together as a group in the parking lot, silently watching as the hearse drives through the gates. As it disappears down the road, we go back inside.

After a few minutes, the residents have forgotten the event. That does not matter. We are entering a new era together. The resident who left is enabling us to care for another. That person has inspired us to find new ways of helping and being together. We have developed as people through the unique connection we had to the resident who is now gone. Every minute with that resident still resonates within us, transforming our minds and our hearts, which will be felt at our care home from here on—there is a ripple effect.

Life at Our Home

We were all sitting in front of the coffin and had just finished singing. One of our oldest residents, Ellen, was very saddened by it and wiped away her tears. She put the napkin down and said, "I guess we're all going to die someday." The staff member sitting next to her took her hand and held it. "Yes, we are. Wasn't that a beautiful song we just sang?" Ellen gave a respectful nod. She agreed it was a nice choice. Then the staff member took a chance and asked her, "What hymn would you like us to sing for you, Ellen?" She answered immediately. *The Sun Is Rising in the East.* (https://hymnary.org/text/the_sun_is_rising_in_the_east)

Let Me Go, Quiet Night

Let me go, quiet Night
Let me stand so still
That those in my care
Sleep, as long as they may
Sleep, as long as they may

Let me wait, winter wind
Wait to let you in
To that room where my calm
Has yet to reside
Has yet to reside

Let me not trample on
A single grain of wheat
Let me see each sprouting seed
Flour, bread—broken in two
Flour, bread—broken in two

Let me love without seeing
What I think I cannot give
Let my doubt be my strength
Take my hope and fill my faith
Take my hope and fill my faith

Like a swallow vanishes
So the night beckons
To rest my head upon your stone
1,000 days are one
1,000 days are one

As small as a bird flying
Unsheltered across the sea
Waves crashing under me
All I've known: all changes
All I've known: all changes

—Jonas Breum

https://www.youtube.com/watch?v=bzhHkLKN0Zg

Just think of how much that soul has given us to share with the next, to someone else who needs to recuperate, to be uplifted, to be welcomed, to regain the will to live. Within days, we begin making preparations for someone new to step inside with their family. Death can also make way for new life.

The day the new resident enters our shared living space, the staff are well-equipped. We are once again prepared and ready to provide that good, person-centered care that we can all attest is the most effective and powerful form of treatment for dementia.

━━━━◆◆◆━━━━

Questions for Reflection

1. Describe what happens in your care home when a resident dies. Does your process allow space for staff, family, and residents to mark the end of the person's life in a respectful way?

2. Although your customs and laws may be different from those at Dagmarsminde, are there ideas presented in this chapter that you would like to implement in your home?

3. The author shares that the resident who has passed away has "inspired us to find new ways of helping and being together." How does your organization share what is learned from working with an individual resident? What are some ways that staff members can develop together?